MW01222858

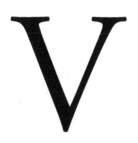

# V

## Zara Fox

**BALBOA**.PRESS

A DIVISION OF HAY HOUSE

Balboa Press books may be ordered through booksellers or by contacting:

Balboa Press
A Division of Hay House
1663 Liberty Drive
Bloomington, IN 47403
www.balboapress.com
844-682-1282

Print information available on the last page.

ISBN: 979-8-7652-3376-4 (sc)
ISBN: 979-8-7652-3378-8 (hc)
ISBN: 979-8-7652-3377-1 (e)

Library of Congress Control Number: 2022915949

Balboa Press rev. date:   11/22/2022

# DEDICATION

To the ones who inspired these chapters and
never turned away from a challenge …
To the ones who knew I would accomplish this and
who supported me all the way through …
You know who you are.
To my Master and to my Sir – you both are the fire
in my life and mean the absolute world to me.
Thank you.

# CONTENTS

Foreword.................................................................. ix

Introduction........................................................... xv

Prologue................................................................. xvii

1  First Time Sinner............................................... 1

2  Viva la Mexico .................................................. 12

3  Tie Me Up........................................................ 32

4  NYE 14-Hour Sex Show ................................... 47

5  Extra, Extra ...................................................... 56

6  Mr. Kink .......................................................... 62

7  Garden of Eve................................................... 69

8  Birthday Boy..................................................... 82

9  Celebration of New Beginnings ....................... 92

10  The Night of DP, DD, or DV ......................... 104

11  Nude Beach Meets The Dungeon ..................... 114

12  Night of the Raccoon...................................... 126

13  Snowflake by Night ........................................ 141

14  Blindfolded by Night ...................................... 150

15  Conscious Mansion party ............................... 160

16  Night of BEhaven ........................................... 172

17    The Night I Went to Paris and London ............................ 182

18    The Vixen's Night of XXXmas Play ................................. 196


Epilogue ...................................................................................... 225

Glossary ...................................................................................... 227

Books .......................................................................................... 243

About the Author ...................................................................... 247

# FOREWORD

If you're looking for a romantic novel with graphic scenes and illicit experiences, one that will knock your socks off and make you say "Whaaa ...?" (I'm imagining a huge grin or a shocked face), I'm going to stop you right here. Maybe this is your book, but if you want something like *Fifty Shades of Grey* by E. L. James, then put this book down and go read *Fifty Shades of Grey*. My book, however, is real, raw, and loaded with experiences. Naturally, names and locations have been changed, and for a very good reason—to maintain confidentiality and protect people's privacy.

Now, with that out of the way, I want you to fully understand why and how I got into "the scene." I had the hunger, the sexual appetite, and the desire to know/learn more about the communities within Canada. Everyone knows the communities are there, but they don't truly know to what extent. There are public events with flashy shows and sex toys aplenty that are more mainstream, such as The Sex Show, and then there are fetish parties in club settings like Sinner's, The Dungeon, Garden of Eve, Lifestyle 101, L'Orange, Aurora, The Oasis, or The X Club—to name a few. In addition to those that are publicized, there are fetish houses with different kinds of rooms, depending on what makes your imagination soar or run wild. In these places, fetish needs are met.

You'll also find that different techniques are practiced in the fetish community, techniques such as rope, fire, electrical, whip, and spank play. Fetish play rarely, if ever, leads to sex; fetish needs, sensations, and desires are met through these kinky outlets where you can find just about anything you fancy. Rope play itself involves all sorts of techniques. It can even be mainstream where it's all about the roper and ropee's connection, feeling the patterns, or expressing a sense of style and technique that takes years of practice to perfect.

From here I'm going to tell you my story, and yes, drugs, sex, and alcohol are involved. I'll start from the beginning, at The Sex Show where there are gadgets galore, pole dancers, demos on display—the works. I still remember "grinder girl"; as the name implies, she has a grinder that she uses on her metal-shielded body, and she grinds the metal cover on her crotch like it's a dildo. The show is almost like a glamorous, high-priced toy fest with fantasy costumes and lessons for the unknowing to feast their eyes on. (I've been there three years in a row—*cough, cough*—and this year I dressed up as a sexy cop.)

To this day, I still remember watching a (BBW) bigger, younger woman (bottoms receive) get spanked with a wooden paddle on stage in front of a live audience until her ass was red. The Top (the person doing the spanking) was graciously talking dirty to the audience, where (to my surprise) this woman's mom was sitting and watching as moans poured out of her daughter's mouth. This level of sexual openness was shocking to me. Mind you, I would never in my right mind do this in front of my mother, and I hope she isn't reading here … Hi, MOM! STOP reading now if you want me to remain the little princess that I am … so, off you go! XO!

Now, on to the games. The Sex Show is where I bought my very first tie-downs and body icing which, I might add, was yummy … but very sticky so I suggest a little shower playtime as well or wipes for clean-up or "after care." I do have honey dust that comes with an application brush. It is very inviting because every time you get kissed or licked, you taste like honey nectar and no mess!.

Along with the nights of club scene drunkenness, I've had my fair share of hitting three-plus clubs in one night, i.e., going to crazy afternoon lunch delights with a DJ and full patio BBQ before later moving on to a rooftop penthouse party, then an evening of dancing at another after-party. I remember looking up at the stars, thinking how wonderful my life was, and having a guy sitting next to me, making sure I had his number. Later, we got chased out of a building we weren't supposed to be in and laughed our way home.

I've been to almost every club where I live, and each one has a class factor, a slutty factor, a friendliness rating, a music rating, and an atmospheric vibe. I'll go back in time to tell you about one "lovely" night in Brick City, where I lived for a couple years. I was rocking my very tight, extremely short black dress, even though I still didn't fully know how to do my makeup and hair. It was a small venue with lots of seating, a mainly bar setting, chandelier lighting glistening everywhere. For a small place, it looked halfway decent. The music was ok at best, and the girls glared at me. *Don't judge me just yet*, I said to myself. I was there with a group of friends, and we ordered drinks: Sex on the Beach for them, and for me, a slim— vodka, water, lime.

After paying for my drinks, I turned around to a random guy— let's call him "Slop" —who was telling a story like an Italian—very expressively—and *crash!* There goes my friend's drink and mine, all down the front of my dress. Fun times … He quickly said sorry and bought us shots to make up for it, in addition to replacing our original drinks—doubled. When I turned away from the bar for the second time, I encountered an angry girl—let's call her "Bee." I simply asked the guy if he knew her. He shook his head and said, "Don't know her." At that, she got even more upset, and when I leaned over to whisper something in his ear, I saw fire in her eyes. She started calling me all sorts of colorful names— "Fucking cunt bitch" and "Wanna go, you slut?!" I quickly realized she was drunk and crazy, so I asked the guy watching next to me if he knew her. Confused, he replied blankly, "No … don't you?!" I said, "Hell no! She just started the crazy train, and I do not want to catch that ride. I want a refund!" Before I could turn away again, she threw her drink down the front of my dress. My only reaction was laughter and a loud, "REALLY!?" I was confused as fuck about why this girl was trying to pick a fight, but I didn't care too much about the extra drink on my dress as my tight black thing was already soaked from the drink that random-guy-number-one had accidently spilled on me.

This was getting out of hand very quickly—the big mouth on her, no one around. Finally, her friend saw what was going on and came up to me, telling me to get off her BFF's boyfriend. I pointed to the guy next to me that I had been flirting with, and she looked confused. She said, "No, no, the guy that bought you a drink." I replied, "OH! You mean the guy who spilled a drink on me and replaced it?" She finally figured out that her friend was crazy and went over to her after telling me sorry. She tried calming her friend down, but I think a stun gun or tranquillizer would have been better.

The spilled drinks had made my dress a little cold, so I found my way to the bathroom. I had to walk past those girls, and the names kept on flowing when I passed the crazy one, let's call her Bee. I didn't care. I had a mission called "I don't give a fuck, I'm cold." Drying off under the air dryer was the only thing on my mind. Who cared about these girls' trippy jealous behavior? I wanted to relax and be dry. In the bathroom, I squeezed out the wet mix of liquors from my—thankfully—black dress. I said to myself, "Thank God, I love black."

After I was somewhat dry, I was now thirsty and really wanted a drink, but when I got about five steps out the door, the damn girl Bee and her friends were there waiting. They said sorry and wanted to talk. I wasn't having any of their shit, so I said, "No worries, but I'm not talking with you guys. I just want to drink right now. Have a great night." Well, apparently, denying a drunk girl's request drives them even crazier, so the place finally decided it was time to drag the five-foot, potty-mouthed girl with no class out. I sighed with relief and sat down to a shot of—*Oh, dear!*—Red Bull and vodka.

One hour and two phone numbers later—one guy even putting his slobbery tongue down my throat while grabbing my ass—I was crashing and hard. I put my head down on the table and suddenly blackout time took over. We got kicked out and walked home. A Skytrain photoshoot along the way with friends was a must. Skytrain parties are always a good time to work on your pole moves and balancing skills, while moving your way back by sitting on strangers' laps and asking them random questions about life while nursing your to-go cup and painting random strangers' nails with the bright pink nail polish you have on hand.

Still with me? Good …

After experiencing many club adventures and different situations, I sometimes wondered how it all escalated so fast. I can say with certainty that I'd rather be somewhere I feel respected, where the environment is friendly and welcoming, and consent is a must. This is what I found at fetish parties and sex-positive events. I felt safer and more at home in a community where that behavior is not tolerated or ignored. That's when I started exploring, researching, and seeking out more experiences, which is what this book is about—my fantasies and sexy times, along with the lessons I learned along the way.

I wished for a lifestyle/kink/sex-positive book, workshop, or even just an open conversation around the shit that can happen. A book on how to find out your kink would have been great too. That's why I've written this book. Not all events are cheery and great with orgy fun that goes smoothly. In this book, I talk about how I found my community, myself, and my inner kink. I also reveal the lessons I learned.

It is my hope that this book will help you understand the growth that comes with exploration as well as help you navigate the hard stuff. This book is also for you if you are looking to explore and understand some basics.

This is the story of how I went from vanilla to Vixen.

Stay safe, stay sexy,
Z

# INTRODUCTION

This book is organized so you can read one chapter at a time: a night of exploration, followed by the lessons I learned after the experience. The asterisk (*) indicates glossary terms that you may or may not know. A glossary will then follow each chapter, and at the end of the book for all. Two asterisks (**) indicate that a term was introduced in another chapter and that the term can also be found in the glossary at the back of the book.

When I first went into the lifestyle, I had no books, no help, and no guidance—except whatever rules were communicated at the place I was at. There was no lifestyle etiquette, no "what to do after this happens," so this book is that!

In the back, you will also find a list of my favorite books that have helped me expand educationally and navigate through life. Maybe they can help you too!

# PROLOGUE

To be honest, I wasn't always into kink ... now that's a lie. When I was little, I made Barbie and Ken perform sexy role play. My friends and I played doctor. After eight years of CCD class, being in a Christian family, and questioning everything, I never understood the limitations. When I was younger, I never understood why my male best friend couldn't sleep over and build a fort with me.

After learning how Mary "magically" got pregnant, I was told it was a miracle. The last time I was in church, I was afraid the holy water would make a red cross on my forehead for my sin of drawing evil clowns on the paper money packets that were used to "grow" the community. My inner life overpowered me, and I didn't know what to do with my thoughts ... I used to draw, write, take on any and all activities that came my way ... until I realized I was never able to find answers to any of my questions, and no one around me had the answers I needed either.

I wondered about my inner desires, my abilities, my soul's calling. I wanted to know how "miracles" could happen or be created. I wanted more and desired more ...

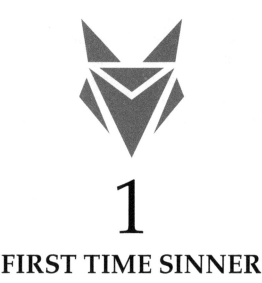

# 1

# FIRST TIME SINNER

~My girlfriend was a free spirit and didn't care who got in her way, when it came to getting her way. She was opinionated and loved to write. Her self-esteem was low, but her drive was high. And her long, black hair adorned her European 5'4" body. She expressed herself without hesitation, not caring who she hurt. It was her world, and she could do whatever she wanted. She was a drinker, that was for sure, and a partier. But I wasn't sure if it was because of me or not. She would always compliment me. My friends said it was out of jealousy, but who knows the full story, since she hid herself well behind an empty wine glass.~

With both nerves and excitement, I gathered three outfits, not exactly knowing what to wear. I had shopped a day prior for costume corsets, fishnet stockings, and booty shorts. I already had the 6" platform stripper shoes that I had purchased while learning pole dancing a while back. Knowing I had much to learn about dancing and style, I shoved everything in a suitcase.

I then quickly slid on a suitable slip dress, for by-passing my parents, and off I went. Turning the tunes on high, to whip up a sexy sense of what was to come, I played "Crazy Bitch" and other songs I had tagged from the strip joints I used to go to on the regular. I was keen to arrive and start drinking my nerves away. And prepping our makeup was a pre-party of its own. It was just two BFFs spilling the beans on life and sex, all while dancing, drinking, and slapping each other's asses. Our makeup slowly transformed from a Picasso-staggered masterpiece to a slick, sexy, chic look.

I slipped my corset on and asked my friend to lace it up gently but tightly. Her hands swiftly smoothed over my back every so often, grazing my baby blonde hairs and tickling me, as she laced up the back of the corset. Lace after lace, sliding through each hole, proved that it was on for the night. But if I was in need of a quick release, there was a hidden zipper on the side; I smirked to myself. As I held my hair up and away from my friend's lingering fingers, I closed my tipsy eyes, wondering what the night would bring. What kind of people would be there? Would I know anyone? Would they all just want to do kinky stuff?

The questions were endless and limitless. My friend knotted the last lace into a triple bow and pressed against me, making me jolt and open my eyes. I bent over, pressed my ass into her, and said, "Spank you." She replied by giggling and slapping my ass. We had that kind of relationship—free, expressive, and aware of each other's boundaries. When we drank, my BFF always pushed the boundaries.

I started chatting about when to leave. And she danced around with a big smile, whipping her hair as if it were a poodle skirt, with a mini camera in her hand. In each other's company, it wasn't uncommon to put on an impromptu photoshoot of some kind. And she always knew to shoot my good side. We danced and downed more shots. I couldn't help but keep wondering what our night would bring. As I turned the music up louder in my friend's bedroom, in her parents' house, I knew very well that we were ready and only had one expectation for the night—to be open.

After checking the time, we chugged our drinks and frantically drunk-dialed for a taxi, while falling over laughing. I took the time to put on two important finishing touches—my black fuzzy handcuffs and black leather spiked collar. And right now, my hair was dyed red, to complement my greenish hazel eyes and pearl-white skin.

We put on our slightly long, oversized jackets to hide our sexy curves from society's eyes. Once at the gate, the bouncer was strict about the dress code. So we flashed him our outfits in order to proceed to the entrance. After entering, we checked our coats. And we were in.

My eyes couldn't stop scanning the room for outfits: PVC, latex, Black Trash Glamour, kinky kitty cats, *puppies* on leashes, and all the hair colors of the rainbow. The common colors were black and red. But there was one exception. It was one couple, and the woman had rainbow everything, from head to toe. Her pink wig caught my eye. We beelined it to the bar, liquid courage to the rescue! As if we needed more, considering how much we'd drank earlier. But flirting with the bartender confirmed that I needed more drunken courage. So I downed a tequila shot for comfort. I then snatched my BFF's hand and started making my way to the dance floor. My gaze instantly took in cages, and I wanted in.

My girlfriend giggled away, as I laughed with excitement. We were dancing as raunchy as ever. And we instantly drew a crowd to us. Three people felt up and down my legs, as I danced and smiled in a heavenly sway. I wanted more, and so did she. Then my girlfriend decided it was time for more drinks, and that was all we needed, as the night progressed. While she ordered us more drinks, I ran to the washroom. The girl in the pink wig was there. Reapplying makeup, she glanced over and smiled.

"There you are," she said. I hurried into the bathroom stall and sat there, wondering what to do. *It's been a while since I've freshened up, do I look OK? What does she want from me?* When I went to wash my hands, she came prancing toward me. Clearly, she was dressed like a unicorn. She wanted to know how I was and if I wanted to play.

"What do you have in mind?" I asked with caution. We were only inches from each other at this point. She grinned, looked me up and down, and her gaze lingered on my lips. I slowly swallowed and looked at her smiling, wondering who would make the first move.

The muffled bass, from the main room outside, was throbbing into the washroom. She and I stared at each other for what seemed to be longer than ten minutes, but it was actually just several tense seconds. She then swept my hair off my shoulder, revealing my neckline and hoop earrings that must have glistened in the florescent light. I took a chance and went in to passionately kiss her, opening her lips wide so our tongues could dance, like lost lovers in the night.

I must have taken her by surprise. My heart began to beat faster, after my head caught up with my actions. My eyes were shut, so I could fully feel her. I then moved my hand from her neck to her hair. I grabbed it, to grasp her even more. I tugged ever so slightly; she smirked and acknowledged my move toward our fantasies. She drew in closer, and I wondered what to do next. And I gasped at her response, knowing very well that I would do what she wanted.

She inhaled sharply, startled by my surprising gesture of dominance. I was curious and even surprised at myself. I wanted to proceed more, and I gently took deep breaths, allowing myself to get lost in the moment. I moved my tender fingers along her well-exposed neckline and her neck, proceeding to her collarbone. I traced the tendrils downward, toward her tender, welcoming breasts. We looked at each other, before glimpsing downward, watching my fingertips tickle her cleavage.

I watched her chest push quickly in and out. It was full, plump, and pushed up by her corset. Her boobs were almost popping out. She then leaned her head back, to give me more room for exploring. Her exposed neck and breasts were mine for the taking, and soon, I was kissing her all over. I soon stopped and realized that we were still in the bathroom, with the bass thumping away. She wanted me to do a mini photoshoot with her, since she could tell I was starting to pull away.

Then reality struck us both when I realized my friend was still waiting for me outside the bathroom. I told her we'd continue later. She replied with a simple, soft, breathless reaction, "You bet ya." Then she started to readjust herself in the mirror and winked at me, and I slapped her juicy ass before I left.

The lighting and dance floor were in full swing, and the club was full of amazing creatures. Even more exciting, my girlfriend had found a cage for us to dance in. We all jumped in and started dancing and grinding against one another, seducing hundreds of onlookers. I used the bars of the cage to keep my drunken balance, while doing never-ending dips to get down low and dirty. And my girlfriend's hands were flailing about.

We had to try and fend off the hands that were trying, some succeeding, to pet us through the bars of our cage. I was getting ready to bite back, but in all honesty, we loved the attention. We loved the atmosphere, which was enhanced by our easy acceptance of every embrace and opportunity to express our sexual prowess that came our way. Getting bored of the cage—*yeah, right*—we decided to explore the rest of the club, since we had yet to venture around.

Everyone had different outfits on and were embracing their own inner vixen and kink* with confidence, no matter what shape, size, ethnicity, race, or sexuality. It was a whole world of just being in the atmosphere, of letting go and feeling the music, of being a fantasy, and of embracing what came your way.

Thinking we knew what we were in for and dancing up a storm, we went to the dance floor. As soon as we got there, I was given a pet on a leash. Not knowing what to do, I just held the leash that was attached to a puppy. Or I should say, *good boy* puppy. All the while, I looked like a lost puppy myself. Fully masked in a puppy play* outfit, he had a muzzle on that resembled a dog's nose. The masked area covered his face in resemblance to a dog as well; the leather brackets went up and over his head, complete with leather ears. His back was braced. Even his paws were leather bound in the form of puppy paws and tail to match. His owner went off momentarily, making me his walker at that moment. He rubbed up against me, wanting me to pet him and dance so I played, scratched his ear, and doggy-danced on the dance floor until his owner came back.

I was half relieved once the pup's owner came back in her all-black latex body suit. The pup was dancing with his ass in the air, rubbing against me, almost as if he were trying to see if I would go further with him. Smiling, I gave the leash over and turned around to a lovely couple, half of which I had previously had fun with in the bathroom. I turned to my friend, and we hustled through the crowd to the stage. There was a crow with feathers and a beak, masked creatures of all kinds, and a DJ booth to top it all off. We started dancing again—*damn right, dirty and grungy*—I expected us to look like drunk, sloppy, bopping girls, but we did get compliments.

After a few hours and becoming drenched in dancing sweat, I longed for water and again proceeded with slight embarrassment to the bartender I had hit on previously. Knowing very well he would not be impressed, I slammed back my water as if it were a shot and ended up choking a bit. That was embarrassing, but at least I made the bartender laugh with my clumsy attempt at getting it all down my throat at the same time.

Making my way back and using my arm as a napkin to wipe the water from my face and chin, I looked up to a couple approaching me. It was the pink-haired woman from earlier; by her man's side this time, she kissed me passionately without hesitation, and I blushed. My girlfriend, jumping with excitement, joined in and we all proceeded to switch between making out, feeling each other up, and dancing in flowing ecstasy. Since I had some experience with girls, but not fully, this was going to be a fun night.

Eventually, the night started dimming and the crowd dissipated. My girlfriend and I were invited back to the couple's place. We looked at each other and gave a slight *You wanna?* look and said, "Why not?"

When we got to the couple's place, a small black cat welcomed us. The place was one big, long hallway underneath a house. Tumbling to the bedroom, I was nervous, but the booze was still helping my courage. I went to the bathroom to freshen up. After washing my face, I looked into the mirror and said, "Well, this is happening."

The couple went straight to the bedroom, knowing exactly what to do and how to proceed. They began before we had even entered the room. My girlfriend jumped on the bed and just lay there till I came out of the bathroom. I had been thinking about what I was about to get myself into. I knew this was another one of my adventures, but it was different than other times as the couple was fully aware of what was going to happen.

We all sat on the bed and started petting each other while the boyfriend mostly watched me go down on his multi-colored girlfriend. He made out with her while he fingered my friend. She moaned and started groping me in the process. Suddenly, it got heated and the boyfriend turned to me and ripped my fishnets open to get to my sopping wet pussy. While I pleasured his woman, she smoked a joint in the process, smiling. I adjusted my position for a better view of his girlfriend's swollen lips. He started licking me and I couldn't help but moan, and that moan transferred to his girlfriend. She reached over and grabbed his hair to push him more into me. I had to grab her hips in order to stay where I was. It was hard to keep pleasing her while I was getting so much enjoyment, so much attention. My girlfriend started playing with the guy's ass. After a few moments, he got up and got his GoPro camera out to take pictures. No faces, only action to be enjoyed by him and his girlfriend for later. I moved over to my girlfriend and started going down on her. She moaned and wiggled, giving me the cues to let me know she was enjoying herself. More and more, her breath came tight and fast. Her pussy throbbed and swelled for more every time I stopped to re-position myself. I noticed she was drunk, tired, and dripping with sweat, but she was able to climax without worry, shame, or guilt. I moved with her swaying hips to keep her going till the end, for when I could taste her satisfied pussy.

I turned around to look at the couple. The guy was grabbing and massaging her breasts with his face engulfed in his girl's clit. He was tongue-fucking her the way she liked it. He went harder and grabbed her hands and pressed them off to the side, making sure she could not move. Her sounds and expressions, through her rosy-fleshed face of sweat, said it all.

The scent and energy in the room was enough. I flipped over for my turn. I realized I had been giving more, and soon I had them both pleasuring me. The woman teased me with her tongue and tickled me gently with her long fingernails, nail polish slightly chipped. She proceeded to tell her boyfriend what to do to me, while biting her lip. I was in sensory overload, not having too much experience but having enough to know just what I like to cum. To my wonderful surprise, he had a tongue ring, and he slid it in and around all the right spots slowly, gently grabbing my hips to move me more into his face and to penetrate me even more, as if it wasn't enough already.

His girlfriend grabbed my hands and placed them so I would stay put. I started to tremble, and thoughts started to pour in. I didn't know what to do. To release or to tense up, to pretend or to turn around, or to please his woman one more time. *Wait, I need to get food tomorrow,* popped into my head. *I need to get my girlfriend home, so her dad doesn't wonder where we've been all night.* Looking around now and noticing the sun was coming up, I decided to kinda fake it by tensing and continuing to moan as I didn't feel comfortable releasing fully in their embrace. She kissed me and said, "Good boy," to her man, and they made out above me.

After two hours of play, no actual penetration except tongue and fingers had occurred. Thinking about it now, I only really went down on the girls. I reached over and woke up my friend who had passed out. We set off into the early morning sun after exchanging

Facebook names in order to keep in contact. She could barely stand up so she leaned into me as I held her, knowing very well she wouldn't remember the whole night. Even to this day, I know I am missing bits and pieces. Calling a cab and not knowing where we were at 5:30 am, we slowly made our way through the streets, tumbling along in our heeled boots. When we got home, we crashed at the first sight of her bed. I lay there, in the afterglow of my first foursome …

## The Lessons

I asked myself after that night what I maybe could have done differently or changed about it in order for me to have felt safer, been more open; I ask myself if I was ok to even have proceeded in the state I was in.

Asking for permission was one thing that arose, and this was not done fully. Consent is a must in these kinds of environments. Yes, I could have said no at any point in the game, but having that open conversation at the starting line makes trusting the situation easier.

Another is having that dreadful I-don't-want-to-but-I-have-to conversation. The conversation of *Are you clean?* and *Do you have protection?* Yes, it might kill the mood for some, but get used to it; the more you ask, the more natural asking becomes. Also, the more sex you have, the more important it is to ask. And not knowing is even worse. Add to that the possibility of catching something that's untreatable, something that you would have to live with for the rest of your life.

Always make sure you are aware of what is happening. For example, taking pictures or videos might not be the best idea, unless you're with someone you trust, someone who wants to share those memories later, moments that you two can watch and appreciate together. It's fun to watch you and your lover having sex. It's kinda hot, too!

You should also wear easy, accessible clothing or things will/

might get ripped. Wearing layers is great if they are easy to get off. If they aren't easy to get off, you're bound to rip or tear things in the moment. Trust me. I have broken a belt buckle, ripped a shirt and a skirt, and even broken things around the bedroom. Which reminds me—if your room is going to be a playroom, please clean up. Sometimes legs and arms or other things might get tossed or stretched or flung around in the heat of the moment. Sorry to everyone whose house I've have been at; I have broken things that have been in my way.

Constantly check in with the group during the play date, not just at the beginning. Yes, it's hard when you're all wrapped up in the moment. You imagine they will just say no if they don't want it, right?! WRONG! Out of respect for everyone involved, check-ins are required. Checking in also keeps everyone happy, and keeps things going, especially when playing with new people. You never know when things might get out of control or if someone doesn't want to speak up. CHECK IN, trust me. Read body language, have a safe word* or action.

Finally, don't drink a ton. Drinking will interfere with your ability to think rationally. Yes, we all do this to calm our nerves so we can be all "loosey-goosey," but there is a downside. You could regret it the next day. Also, your mind disconnects more with every drink you down. Stick to a limit, and your mind, gut, and body will like you so much more. Plus, your sensibilities will be better once you're sober.

## Glossary

*Kink*: Something that brings you pleasure/turns you on but also bends away from the "straight and narrow." You could have a kink for bondage, whips, chains, dress up, role play, or something more subtle. Kinks are usually considered non-conventional sexual practices.

*Play*: A term I use that includes everything up to oral, but not penis-in-vagina. "Play" could mean different things for different people, so ask!

*Puppy Play or Pup Play*: This term is for a situation in which one person takes on the role of a pup, while the other one takes on the role of a handler, consensually of course.

*Safe Word*: A word, usually other than "no," that indicates a stop to everything and/or that a check-in is needed. This can also be a gesture or something you do, such as dropping something in order to signal to a play partner that they need to stop. Sometimes, words won't compute or are limited by a gag or some other element in a scene.

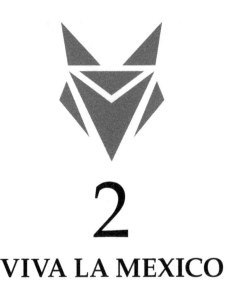

# 2

# VIVA LA MEXICO

~He was charming and handsome and said all the right things. He spoke the language and spun me around the dance floor. He knew salsa, and that meant that he knew how to sway his hips. His blond hair and hazel eyes were trouble from the start. I fell for a boy who was getting married, and yes, that meant I crashed his bachelor party, bienvenidos Max.~

A dear friend of mine wanted to go on vacation. She wanted a crew of us to go. Three of us could afford to bounce. She shopped for deals and booked it within the week. My excitement was escalating. I was ecstatic and relieved at the idea of going on vacation before Christmas. We were best friends who, back in the day, went clubbing every weekend to the famous Illusions out in Midtown. We knew how to party—all too well. So why not go on an all-inclusive trip together … naturally!

Once on the flight, we just knew it was going to be an epic

adventure. After checking out the resort, we saw that our hotel had a nightclub on site. Singing and gossiping to no end along the way, we decided what adventures we would partake in once there. Upon arrival, the warm exotic air hit my face. I couldn't help but close my eyes and smile in the intense heat that covered my pale, white skin.

The resort was gorgeous. Marble throughout the halls, and near the entrance, a water fountain with a statue of a half-naked lady, covered in what looked like sheets. In the garden area, the grass was very green, and the walkways were lined with red pebbles. There was another water feature, a gazebo bar at its center. Excited to explore the resort and the beach front, we proceeded to our room, drinks in hand. When we entered our room, we immediately took in more marble and two beds in a light beige, peach-orange color scheme, like the rest of the hotel. The open washroom was large enough to literally dance in; in my head, I said a silent, *Thank God*, because there was a door to the toilet. I was relieved that there was privacy, as there was only a shower curtain closing off the shower from the rest of the room. In the corner of my eye, I saw the bar; it was a full bar with all the hard but delicious nectar we could possibly want on our tongues. I smiled, thinking about how much trouble this could all be.

Once settled into the room, I instantly heard our neighbors on their balcony, and my girlfriend showed signs of shyness for the first time. She was quiet, not wanting to show or introduce herself, which was unlike her. I moved to the balcony, rolling my eyes at her silliness. While checking out the view, I got the chance to introduce myself to our neighbors. To my surprise, they were our age; two guys, one girl, which was the opposite of our crew of two girls, one guy. I couldn't not laugh at that. I went into play mode. We were starving as we'd only had a drink at the airport and a dollar beer on the bus ride over, after being called gringos. We scoped out the swim-up pool bars and dinner places to find the best spot.

We ate, drank, and then drank some more from the full bar in our room, keeping company with the curious geckos that made their way in. We were already in full swing, hitting up the pool, taking in the oceanic view, and enjoying the open bar. We were tired but decided to chill that night and explore what the hotel had to offer.

My best friend and I chilled as my guy friend—let's call him "Mike"; he was my GF's ex back home— wanted to explore and find some Mary Jane to smoke. My girlfriend wouldn't stop talking about her boyfriend back home; she wanted to email him at the café before bed. Thinking it would only take a few minutes, I agreed to go. We saw that the drunk scene was in full swing, and the nightly entertainment was right outside our balcony. After going to the bar, I sat waiting, not wanting to connect to society while I was away. I believed in disconnecting from electronics on holidays; others not so much.

Mike was getting bored and decided to hit on me while I drank my Long Island Iced Tea. Since I hadn't seen the drink list, I asked for a standard one. Laughing, we flirted a little too far. Mike kissed my neck and moved his hands closer to my crotch. At that point, I pushed him away. He decided to bounce to go see what other trouble might await him that night. Now on my second drink, I wanted to leave too, so I asked my friend how long she would be. Every so often, I would look over to see if she was finishing up; she replied as if I was annoying her, "In just a bit, but you can go if you want."

I had thought we were on vacation together to have fun and explore, but she must have had another agenda, which was okay as it was only the first night. I decided to finish my drink and chat with the people sitting beside me. They were drunk out of their minds. I couldn't help but laugh at what they were trying to pull with me, sluggishly putting their arm around me and slipping, almost falling over while I remained upright on my stool.

While my friend was typing away, one of our neighbors walked in—Tammy. She sat down with my girlfriend. I had thought my girlfriend was just checking in with her BF since she'd just arrived. When I went over to her, she said she was gonna stay with Tammy. I looked at them both and said I would go to the room then. Taking my drink to go, I wandered around the hotel and went down to the ocean to catch a glimpse of the waves crashing on the sandy beach. I buried my feet in the still slightly-warm sand.

After meandering slowly to our room, I crashed on the bed and stripped awkwardly while looking up at the ceiling. Impressively, I did not spill my drink. I then proceeded to top off my drink at the quick access bar with a glass push tab and decided it was game on.

I put on some music and headed into the shower. To my surprise, I was a little tipsy and enjoyed the sensation of water dripping all over my tender body, its purity still untouched by the sun. Running my fingers through my hair, I heard the door shut, suddenly stopped what I was doing, and nervously said, "Hello?"

Mike greeted me back and suggested he join me in the shower. Laughing, I said, "You wish!" in a very *try me* way. When I realized I was the naked one, my eyes widened, and I frantically reached for my shirt. I quickly put it on and toweled up my hair up just before he could try something. I opened the curtain as he approached and totally teased him. He stopped me in my tracks; I moved … he moved with me. Then he graciously let me pass with a bowing gesture.

I swiftly moved, my head held high as if I'd won, and I was the queen. Suddenly, he pushed me onto the bed, laughing. I was startled so he stopped and asked where our friend Linna was. I told him that she still wasn't back from the computer she was glued to. He made himself a shot of tequila and so did I. We knocked them back, and I plopped fully on the bed, lying back with the lights off. The room spun just a tad; maybe it was the booze, maybe the lack of food, maybe the heat, or all of above. But I was feeling playful. Mike joined me in bed and chatted as he started touching my body, trying to tempt me, tickling my senses, seeing what he could get away with. He kissed my neck as I lay there half-sleeping after our chat and half-buzzed out of my mind. I closed my eyes and just concentrated on the feeling. I hadn't gotten any in a while, so I was craving touch, motion, energy, and I started to embrace it.

He slowly moved his fingertip, gliding closer and closer towards my outer lips, just grazing them to tease me. I moved closer to him, my eyes still closed. Wanting a kiss, he brushed my lips. I knew he could feel my heart beat when he let out a pleased sigh. He moved in then, kissing my neck and grabbing my ass as if he didn't need to ask. He moved my ass up against his crotch, pressing me against his hard cock. I smiled. Making someone go instantly rock hard turned me on. I gently pushed my ass into him, feeling his pulsing dick get harder. He grabbed my hips even harder and groaned for more. I let him grab my inner thighs and I tipped my head back with pleasure, not fully registering the situation—just allowing it. His hand migrated down towards my clit, swirling in my gushing juices. Soon, I realized how much I'd missed a man, missed and longed for everything; the touch, the warmth, the energy. He glided his fingers in and around, using my own lubrication. I was breathing heavy now and wanting more.

Still entangled in only the sensation and detached from any emotion thanks to the drinking, I turned around and we started kissing. His lips, plump, full, and moist, knew where to lead a kiss. I let him. Mike lifted my shirt to feel my breasts and worked his way down to my throbbing clit. I wanted his tongue. He lifted the covers to proceed in worshiping my cunt.

Kissing, licking, teasing, his long tongue performed one stroke at a time, making my hips move up towards his face for more. He laughed when I moved his head back down. He was undeniably good at what he did; either that, or my detachment from it all made it so right. With every slow-motion flick, I moaned, wanting more. He then started to tongue fuck me while switching it up with his fingers from my clit to my pussy. I couldn't handle it and moaned my release with my back arched and my head held back. After I realized what had just happened, he came back up, wiping my yummy juices from his face. He commented that I tasted good, a little sweet, and all I could say in my head was *umm interesting* and *cool*. He cuddled with me, pressing his still-erect cock into my thigh-gap area. The door swung open at the same time I realized that I didn't want to have sex with him. Linna had finally come back. "Fuck, guys, it's hot in here," she said.

"Oh, yeah, sorry. Forgot to turn on the AC," Mike said, knowing very well it was our lust that had made it so. I pretended to sleep. Well, half-pretended as at this point, I was going to fall asleep from over-exhaustion. As we said our goodnights, I wondered if I'd just dreamt what had happened.

The next day was gorgeous and to my surprise, everything was the same. We hustled down to the pool for our morning brecky and drink. Then off to the water we went. We were finally starting our seven-day suntan adventure and relaxation. Linna needed to go to the bathroom, where she ran into our neighbors on their way to have lunch, so she said bye and joined them. I wasn't hungry at that point so me and Mike moved the long chairs two meters closer to the water and went back and forth between relaxing in the sun to wave surfing on boogey boards.

Linna was gone for a while, and I started to get nervous, so I left Mike by the water and went to the room, where I found a very angry note stating how Mike and I were bad friends for leaving her on her own. She also said she was going to be at the beach. We were just there. Maybe she hadn't seen us because we'd been in the water cooling off, but our stuff was on the chairs still. I went back to the ocean but still hadn't seen her by 5:00 pm. I went over to the chairs and asked Mike to start looking. He found her and she started yelling at us, saying, "Where the hell were you?" and "If I'd known you two were together, I would have never come!" to "I thought we were here together." I tried to rationalize with her but was unsuccessful. I told her we were all together, that Mike and I were not together. I didn't understand why she was getting so upset over nothing. "We tried looking and couldn't find you," we both told her in exasperated tones.

Linna didn't believe us and called me a liar. At that point, I'd had enough; no one calls me a liar, and for all I knew, she hadn't looked for us either, but I'd taken her word for it. I said, "I'm done!" to her and that I wasn't responsible for her and her happiness. I started to leave and so did Mike. I stopped after realizing that I hated being mad even though she was clearly upset for other unknown, underlying reasons. I turned back and sat next to her. Linna said, "I thought you were done with me." She cried and rolled her angry eyes at me. I told her I wouldn't leave a friend over something so silly. She still wasn't impressed. I told her we could agree to disagree since she clearly wasn't going to acknowledge that I was right.

We sat there and calmed down, then I went to grab us more drinks. I grabbed margaritas with a twist while I got hit on by a guy in the pool next to me. I told him I had to run to my friend and hustled the drink over to her. Then the neighbors showed up. Linna acted super nice to everyone except me. I soon realized I was out of place, so I said I was going to the pool if she was ok with it. She replied with a simple, "Yeah, go," not even looking at me. Again, I asked her if it was cool. She said, "Of course," with a curled lip. I knew she wasn't ok, but she wouldn't express it, and I wasn't about to get swept up in more drama on a holiday.

I proceeded to the pool since the guy I had been talking to earlier was still there. He was expressive and full of energy; he told me he was a vegan and that he was well-traveled. I could tell he had a way with women. His charm and ease made it easy for me to approach him. There was something about him that intrigued me. I didn't know what it was, but I wanted to find out. His blond hair, hazel eyes, and chiseled body made him easy on the eyes, and his casual attitude of anything goes was exciting and mysterious at the same time.

The conversation progressed through the usual: Where do you work? What do you do? Where have you traveled? What are your goals? Blah blah blah … I drank and drank, and we got closer and closer. He told me that he'd been living in Mexico for over a year, bouncing around from resort to resort until he got kicked out of the country. This was his first trip back since. He told me about resort life and how he would get a group in a circle to massage each other's shoulders and go lower and lower, and then say, "Nah, ah ha! Don't be handsy! Not that low, you horny gringos." We also talked about his diet, since I'd asked how he kept his figure rock hard. Being vegan and a taekwondo instructor helped a lot. To me, that was sexy, like he had a hidden ninja strength in him.

He wanted to walk around and invited me to join him. I thought about telling my friend but decided she was ok with the others. She also didn't seem all that stoked about hanging out with me. I moved off his lap and grabbed us to-go drinks for our walk. He wanted to grab a snack from his room, and all I thought was, *Cool, I get to see his room.* When we passed by the beach, he asked the guy in charge about going jet skiing. The guy said it'd be free in an hour. He looked at me and asked if I'd be down; he didn't have to ask twice. Of course I was! Open ocean, Mexico, jet skiing … Can you say, "Hell yeah"?!

I remembered our neighbor-friend Tammy wanting to go as well, so I asked her, and Max asked his friend. She was wide-eyed with excitement. "OMG yes! With who?! Do I have to do anything for it?" I laughed. "No, it's just for fun. Leave it to me." I winked at her.

Linna looked at me with disgust and anger. She said, "Why didn't you ask me?" "I didn't know you wanted to," I said. "Tammy had mentioned being interested before." All she said was, "Oh, ok" before turning around and putting in her ear plugs again. I didn't want to get wrapped up in her passive-aggressive antics since I believe in saying what you want and expressing it clearly, or at least discussing it, not just keeping it all in. I wanted to take away her anger and her sensitivity, but I couldn't; she had to learn to do that on her own—me holding her hand was not going to teach her anything.

When I went with Max to his room, he threw me on to the bed. Now that I understood the situation, I pulled him towards me. He said, "Hold your horses." I needed a snack, so I said, "Oh! You are actually hungry for food, aren't you?" I smirked, and he smiled at the open language I was already using with him. He snacked, and I finished my drink. I decided to make another in the full bar he had in his room. When I turned around, drink in my hand, he was already relaxing on his bed. I put my drink down and climbed over him so that I could relax next to him. He stopped me, pulling me on top of him.

He kissed my neck and grabbed my face to give me a luscious kiss on my parted lips. We tasted like margarita and fruit. It was perfect. He flipped me over so he was on top of me and offered to give me a massage. Delighted, I lay flat while he got to know my body, kissing and teasing along the way. He brought out lotion from the bathroom and massaged me with it from head to toe. He snapped my bathing suit straps and teased about it being in the way, so I took off my top. I felt his dick getting hard on my ass while he calmly and smoothly massaged my shoulders. I knew he was getting more and more aroused because his movements were faster and more staggered down my shoulder blades. When he got to my ass, he slowed down. I knew he was admiring how plump it was. He said, "You could bounce a quarter off this, couldn't you?" I said, "Probably."

"One sec," he said as he grabbed a quarter and bounced it off my ass. I blushed as we both laughed. I wanted to turn around and kiss him, but he was having none of it. He turned me around and slapped my hands down on either side of my body in the process. Crouching down, he whispered in my ear, "I'm not done yet." I closed my eyes in anticipation, and the warmth of his breath, even in this heat, took me by surprise. He proceeded to kiss me all down my back, side to side, pulling down my bottoms for easier access. "Aren't those restrictive?" he asked. I lifted my ass so he could more easily remove them. Kissing and using his tongue to tease me, he stopped short of fully engulfing himself in my throbbing vagina. I was just longing for his next move.

He moved up, gliding his now fully erect dick up my exposed body. He still had his shorts on, so I said sheepishly, "How come

I'm naked and you're not?" He smirked. "Would you like me to be?" I smiled and said, "Aren't those restrictive?" He smirked at my smart-ass attitude and slid them off. His cock slid over my ass as he cradled me. I was wet and ready from his massage, now with a more appropriate tool. I wanted him but didn't want to show that too much as I felt it wasn't my place. He turned me over and started kissing me. We were a hot, sweaty mess at this point. The lotion he'd used made us into a slip and slide. I wanted him in me. I slid my hands down below, but he made a gesture, indicating I was in trouble. He grabbed my legs and cradled my butt so he could better get to my sopping pussy. He licked and fingered, and licked around some more, touching my clit to my outer labia, slithering his way back in. He played with my butt, licking slow, soft then fast; it was a different sensation altogether.

I looked out the sliding glass door at the clear blue sky before closing my eyes to concentrate on the knee-jerk sexual encounter I was having. I was reaching climax; I couldn't help but want more and more. Grabbing the sheets, I moaned, shook, and let out a gasp. I knew he was satisfied with himself for pleasing me. He crawled up, wiped his mouth on the sheets, and started making out with me. I was wet and ready, but tight; I guided him in. Slowly, he penetrated me, inch by inch. I could tell by his face that my pussy felt great to him, and he was trying hard not to blow his load so quickly. He flipped me over so I was on my stomach, and he could fuck me from behind. Since we were sliding everywhere, dripping wet from sweat, it was nice to finish quickly. We both wanted to shower. He went first as I cleaned up, and then I heard the door. To his surprise, I ran into the shower and told him his friends were here. They were loud and turned on music. I listened to them talk about their encounters with women. They obviously didn't know I was in the shower with Max. We kept going because he got hard again when I rubbed his wet body. I wanted him bad! I turned around in the small, cramped shower and glided him into my still-wet pussy. I pressed against the walls for support. He slid right in. The music stopped, and I heard his buddy ask, "Max, do you have a visitor?" I looked out from the curtain and said, "Oh, hey," before pulling it closed again. They laughed and said you better be using protection. We shrugged it off, feeling blurry and dreamy at the same time. They left, and we finished quietly. He pressed his hands to my mouth to muffle the noises I was making and grabbed me even closer.

We dried off and went back downstairs to the jet skis where we met up with his friend from the room and my neighbor, Tammy. On the jet skis, we whipped around like idiots, screaming and yelling and almost hitting each other. Max's jet stalled for a bit, and my top had slipped down. I flashed everyone on the beach while I stood up on the back end of the jet ski, my arms held high. I looked down and didn't care, only making sure I didn't lose it so I was able to pull it up eventually. Our adrenaline was pumping. Afterwards, we all went for a snack and to get some more booze from the room. Tammy and Tim, Max's friend, went to the balcony to chill and chat as Max and I took the opportunity to get down in the sheets again. Tim walked in, turned around, and shut the sliding glass door. He chatted up Tammy some more. Soon, she was going down on him. We figured this out when we heard sounds of pleasure coming from the balcony. We also heard a loud crash—from a chair. Tammy came running in and grabbed me to leave. She was flushed and her hair was out of whack. She looked as if she'd just thrown her clothes on. "Are you alright?" I asked her. Weary and impatient, all she said was, "Let's go." I was naked so I told her to hold on a sec; I needed clothes. She said, "Wow! You got balls," to me as she hovered by the doorway. I took it as a compliment and told Max I'd see him later.

Tammy grabbed my hand immediately after I put on my suit, and out we ran. I didn't know why or what we were running from. "What the fuck happened?" I asked. She told me she shouldn't have done what she did, but what's done is done. I told her there was no shame in this, that she shouldn't feel bad. I could tell she didn't want to talk about it so I dropped the conversation and went to rejoin everyone at the beach. We all set off for dinner.

We decided to go clubbing that night and dang, was I ready. I wanted to dance the night away like last time. We showered, dressed up, and walked over to the club on site. The club smelled of piss and old booze, but after a few drinks, you barely even noticed. The floor was concrete and small, and the locals would come and take over the club on weekends.

I met Andrew and started speaking Spanish with him and his friends. Linna was dancing with the neighbors again. I made new friends quickly and didn't realize Linna had left until later when I went to the washroom and saw them sitting around a table. I told Andrew I would be back. He had called me beautiful in Spanish. I hurried over to my friends, and to my surprise, Max was there too. Everyone was just chilling and chatting.

When I arrived, Linna said, "Ok, see ya!" I replied, "I hope you're not leaving on my account." She fumbled and said, "No, we want to go on the computers for a bit." She was on them every night, sometimes during the daytime as well, talking to her boyfriend. I agreed to join her and Tammy. Max came along to chat with me. I said goodnight to my Mexican friends, surprised at how much Spanish I had remembered; I think it was the tequila.

We stopped at the café to get some well-deserved nachos to snack on. Since I had danced up a storm, and drank so much, I figured I needed to eat something. Tammy and Linna were chatting quietly. I got the impression I wasn't wanted. Tammy had no idea. Max was tired and was going to head to his room so I asked if I could join him. Linna and Tammy were going to be on the computer for a while. I said my farewells for the night. On the way to his room, we decided to take a detour and found a spot with minimal light so we could look up at the stars in the night sky. They were mesmerizing. We lay down for barely five minutes when he moved in to kiss me. I sighed and said, "Wait, what if someone comes?" I looked side to side. He replied, "What people?" "Ahh, touché," I said. He put his hand down my skirt, fingering me slowly at first and then aggressively after my kisses became more aggressive. He pulled his board shorts down and penetrated me again, this time without going slowly; he just took me under the stars as I looked up at the sky. I held him close, trying to avoid making it more intimate by looking into his eyes.

People were coming and going; we would just stand still while they passed, pretending we were star gazing. Then we'd laugh and keep going. I realized he'd lost his nose ring so we searched for it until we saw a guard and made a run for it. Frisky, groping each other, we sped up the stairs, kissing sloppily. Looking around for where to go next, I saw a random door open. I looked inside and gestured for him to come in. It was the laundry room, full of white sheets, towels, and blankets from floor to ceiling. What an amazing opportunity. He asked if this was a good idea. I didn't know, but I said, "Come on ... you scared? Come and get it." He passionately, or drunkenly, pushed me in and up against the metal shelving. I turned around and lifted my silky baby blue dress up invitingly. He pulled his pants halfway down and tried to glide his dick in. It was awkward so I bent down. I looked around, and he suggested the concrete ledge where the laundry was thrown down—basically, the exposed shoot. Unable to see the bottom, I looked at him, scared, and said, "Don't you thrust me over the edge now!" I bent over it and held on, making my body cling to the cement opening. He pressed my hands in his, and I felt his hot, heavy breath against my ear as he thrusted harder and harder inside me. I liked the thrill, the excitement, the adventure. Knowing anyone could come in at any moment was turning me on. His groans told me he was about to cum, and he placed his fingers to my clit, trying to pleasure me. I bit my lip to keep quiet and crouched into his solid figure. I was about to cum when he pulled out and came all over a stack of sheets next to us. I suggested he could have at least picked one. While resting his head on the metal shelving, he acknowledged my logic. Out of breath and legs locking up from making hip thrusting motions with him, I fell to the floor. Then we heard someone or something. We quickly dressed and booked it downstairs to his room.

We quietly opened the door because his roommates were asleep.

Then we crashed in bed. Three hours later, we woke up to his roommate puking and more. For the rest of the night, I covered my face with the sheets in order to avoid the stench that filled the room.

I'd heard rumors circulating around the hotel about a woman getting assaulted in the elevator the night before, so I buckled down and held out until daylight. I kissed Max good morning and goodbye for the day. Making my way back to my room, I said, "Buenos dias," to the janitor after he smiled at me. I figured he knew what I'd been up to. I snuck in and passed out for a few more hours.

Then we were up, wanting to embark on our adventures: going into town one day, then all-inclusive zip lining, water sliding on "the world's biggest, steepest slide," riding farting donkeys, off-roading, hiking, and even a waterfall to line drop from.

After not having seen Mike for a while, and Linna always wanting to sleep early at night, it was nice to reunite. Then the night came once again, and it was game on. Purchasing a club crawl, we were off with 15 others to a zoo bar, a cow bar where they set cinnamon on fire, and then our favorite, a club with an LED-lit floor and bar where we drank the night away. I cried on the beach boardwalk that night after having drunk a lot, since I knew I was losing Linna, and she was acting like it was all ok. I hated fake, and it made me upset. Even though she reassured me, I knew our friendship was still on the rocks. We danced, sang, and hugged, and on the way back, Linna and Mike raced in the bus's upper luggage hold. They crawled from the back to the front after saying they would kick each other's asses and hazing each other. The guide kept saying this was the first time he'd had this happen.

The next morning we lay in the sun, played volleyball, and decided to go to the club in the hotel. Everyone met up from the club crawl. That night was a night of thrilling, adventurous fun. Once night was upon us, we hustled to dress to impress, me in my flowy shirt and tank, my girlfriend in a dress. Bouncing off the walls with excitement, we proceeded to the bar. Linna got us Viva la Mexico tequilas. They were our drink of choice this holiday, and deadly, as you couldn't taste the tequila, only the fizzy juice. You were supposed to place your hand on top of the glass, slam it down three times, and shoot it. Hitting on the guys across the bar and beside us, we made friends quickly as we ordered every drink imaginable, all colors and liquors. After drowning our taste buds, we decided it was clubbing time, and I stole a guy's hat from across the way. We got on top of the tables and started putting on a sexy dance show for the guys. They hooted and hollered, placing dollar bills in our skirts. After almost falling off the wobbly table, it was time to head in for more dancing … after one more drink.

Once inside, the smell wasn't as bad this time because I could smell my own breath of juicy goodness. We danced the night away to "Su Vasa, Who Likes to Party," but my friend was getting bored so she danced with another friend. Max grabbed me, showing off his salsa moves, swaying me around as I staggered, trying to follow his lead. It made me fall in love with the dance, and even more with the boy. But was it love or just infatuation? Or even the drinking and environment we were in?

Max asked if I had a background in dance. I chuckled; I always get asked that. I said I just knew how to move my hips. Then he wanted to lift me, which was great until he slipped. Good thing I didn't get a concussion or anything, just a nice bump on the head. The alcohol I'd ingested helped with the pain, or the pain that should have been there. It was time for another drink. Everyone gave Max hell for dropping me, and they all helped my drunk ass up. Apologizing profusely, Max asked me what he could do. I sheepishly said he could make it up in other ways and winked at him.

Downing another drink was a must and getting some fresh air was another necessity. We got some time to ourselves, which was nice since we still couldn't keep our hands off each other. I looked around and grabbed his arm, leading him to the nearest cabana. "Open air bed, restricted" was posted on the outside. Sheer curtains hid, or rather, didn't hide what went on inside. Sneaking in and looking around, we laughed and pushed each other on top of the table. Trying to be sneaky and quiet was, as you can image, difficult for two sloppy drunks, but it was easy for me to just take off my lace underwear and for him to unzip. Breath heavy, hearts racing, we were constantly in stop-and-go mode so as not to get caught. The table/bed would creek as we rocked back and forth together. We stopped for a moment, wondering if it would collapse on us, then looked at each other and said screw it. Max was trying to hold on to the awkward table to help him out when we heard screaming from the club. We stopped to look around. "If we are still, they might not see us," I said, thinking they were predator animals on the prowl, and drunk ones at that.

After a split second, we heard the pack of animals running full speed to the ocean. We were still keeping a low profile to avoid being seen. Confused, we eventually decided to see what the heck was going on. We opened the curtain and huddled so we could peep through towards the beach. Pieces of clothing were strewn on the sand, a meter away from our feet. We peered down to the dark ocean and smiled at each other before deciding to get a closer look. We walked towards the darkness, accompanied by the crisp warm air and the sound of waves crashing in the distance.

The closer we got, the more clothes we saw. I realized that I recognized the clothes; they belonged to our group of friends. I was in awe. Max looked at me with amazement when I started to strip down. "They're our friends, scaredy cat," I teased. He smiled and started stripping down himself. We ran to join them. The girls screamed before realizing who was joining them. I yelled, "It's me, drunks!" When they heard my voice, they laughed and asked where we'd come from. Max and I said, "Somewhere," simultaneously and smiled sheepishly. We kept our secrets hidden. The girls pestered me for more, but I wouldn't budge. They swam closer, except for the ones that were having a bit too much fun; I could see splashing and hear laughing.

I wanted to do just that, so I started moving further into the darkness. Max followed, splashing me in the process. Trying to be quiet so the guards wouldn't catch us, we fumbled in the waves. I said, "The movies make this look easy." I was out of breath, waves crashing in my face. I spat out water and doggy-paddled back into calmer water so I could toe-touch the shore. The rest of the crew got out and got dressed while I stayed behind with Max to pick up where we had left off. We soon realized the dark water wasn't easy to navigate and interfered with our flow, so we decided to explore somewhere else. I only put on my skirt and top because he had tucked my underwear into his pocket.

*Men have it easy. They only need shorts*, I thought. We rolled around in the sand for only a moment, as it itched like sandpaper, so we switched to one of the white lawn chairs sprawled along the shore, awaiting daylight.

Massaging and kissing in sweet drunken bliss, to my surprise, we saw another couple doing the exact same thing. We figured they wouldn't see us if we stayed still since it had worked last time. There was a shadow under their lawn chair, and when we looked closer, there was a guy laying underneath, pleasuring himself on their account. The couple didn't see because he had positioned himself so he wouldn't be seen. The couple also probably had their eyes closed in bliss. After realizing they weren't going to notice, we stopped to watch for a bit, then moved towards them. The guy shuffled, and they saw him. A fight ensued. We quickly moved, finding another area that had grass. Sex on the beach was definitely on my bucket list.

The patch of grass we'd found between the tennis court fence and the garden had to suffice. It was great riding him while he reached around to double please me. I bit him on the shoulder, trying to muffle my sounds but still get off. He kept telling me, "Down, tiger," because I kept scratching and biting with pleasure. I heard shuffling so I stopped. Max said I was paranoid, but I still stopped every so often while I rode him. I gripped the tennis court fence and squatted over him. His expression told me he was trying not to let go.

Getting caught was not on our agenda. I saw a light in the

distance, and as it moved towards us, we quickly got up, pretending nothing had happened. We were just two lovers in the night, making out passionately. They didn't buy it and radioed in more guards. My heart raced as they were reading out the rules and the fines. In Spanish, we said we were on our honeymoon and that my ring was being re-sized, while holding hands. We protested when the guard started to report his location. We could get fined and kicked out … among other things. When the guard wasn't looking, I ran and hid underneath a chair on the beach. It must have been 5:00 am. The guard radioed in, trying to find me, and then I heard my boy say my name, looking for me. I was torn. My heart throbbed, racing with fear and tension. I waited for the guard to leave and ran hard to the men's room. I was in the staircase when I heard my name and saw Max. Like a reverse, fucked-up Romeo and Juliet, he was looking down from the top floor, calling my name. I ran to him, and he ran to me. The guard caught up just to make sure I was going to bed. He asked if I'd found my husband. I pointed upward and said thank you. Both of us panting, I threw my arms around Max. He picked me up and fiercely kissed me with no filter or hesitation. He lowered me, grabbed my arm, and booked it back to his room.

The next morning, he didn't chat with me and seemed distant. I would ask him where he was, and he would respond, "Umm, with my friends," in an awkward way. I soon realized what was happening; I was a vacation fling. I asked him for his number, and he said he didn't think that was a good idea. While walking back from the club, I asked him why not. He didn't say anything so I asked if he had a girlfriend. Nothing. Startled at his expression, I asked, "Do you have a fiancée?" Again, he didn't say a damn thing … I slapped him and yelled, "If you truly loved her, you wouldn't have been with me in the first place." I ran to my room.

Crying and frustrated, I opened the room to Linna and the neighbor girl sleeping in the bed that I was supposed to be in. Mike was in the other. I realized I hadn't seen him the rest of the trip but was glad he was alive and well. When I crept in, he asked what was wrong. I told him what had happened, and he cuddled me, showing compassion and empathy—when my friend Linna had not. Even on our way back home, she was cold …

## The Lessons

First off, when you go on vacation with friends, make sure you're in the same headspace regarding intentions, and if not, communicate your intentions. After this trip, we were no longer friends. I did run into Max again six months later. He and his fiancée were no longer together so we decided to have a fling back home. Mind you, he did have to go down on one knee and beg me for forgiveness, *wahahahaa!*

Fooling around with a friend, mind you, your girlfriend's ex—in my case, Mike—is a bad idea all around, even if they'd broken up for a good reason. One of the reasons they'd broken up was that my girlfriend was constantly cheating on him. FYI, she doesn't talk to me anymore. However, I did respect her wish of no sex. Yes, it's a free for all, but that doesn't necessarily mean for you. Live and learn and trust your internal guide.

Asking questions before having sex is a must! And please don't assume anything, as it just leads to trouble. Even though he should have mentioned he had someone back home, it's up to you to be in charge of your own life. Remember to put the oxygen mask on yourself first.

Before you have sex, make sure you don't miss out on the most important baby defense of all: condoms. Even if you are on birth control, if you missed a day or are off by half a day, it can screw with your cycle. The best birth control method is to use a condom, but neither are 100% protection so the more, the merrier in this case.

Yes, THE talk about STIs* and such didn't happen from what I remember, and yes, I did get checked out back home, but that was not a game I wanted to play. Play safe!

Yes, there are a lot of things I did on this trip that were about lacking connection to myself because of drinking. Maybe "getting it on" in Mexico, out in the open and getting caught by the guards and almost getting kicked out, not to mention fined, wasn't the best idea. But when you're only thinking of one thing and looking for a thrill … let's just say be careful and trust your gut.

Needless to say, I did get to check a few items off my bucket list!

## Glossary

*STIs*: Sexually transmitted diseases, yay! Not really. They are caused by one person passing on a bacteria, virus, or parasite to another, either during sex or intimate contact. It is best to use protection like condoms when engaging in sexual activities. Some of the most common STIs are: Chlamydia, Gonorrhea, Hepatitis B (HBV), Herpes (HSV-1, HSV-2), Genital warts/Human Papillomavirus (HPV) infection, and Syphilis. For more information, you can always do a good ol' Google search on a reputable site, such as the Mayo Clinic or the Center for Disease Control in your area.

# 3

## TIE ME UP

~I had always been intrigued by the idea of being tied up, and I wanted to explore it more. Maybe rope had been my fetish all along … His genuine smile, empathetic way, and desire to please cried out to me … I could feel his hurt, his pain.~

*J* got invited by my friend "Neil," who'd been wanting to introduce me to the rope scene* for a while. I had met him during my third Halloween Sinner's party. He was a gentle soul and a gentleman. It was 3:00 am; I was outside looking for my friends who had apparently abandoned me by the night's end. I was wearing a black-and-white dancer girl outfit that I'd made from a corset, mini-hat, striped leggings, black garter, and hooker heels; I'd taken a trip to FABrix to hot glue the rest. My hair was all done up to one side, my hat fixed with a white feather, and sheer black drape mesh hung over my exposed side. I looked like a seductive, vintage circus dancer.

I was waiting outside in the dreary wet Ontario weather when he pulled up and asked if I needed a ride. After getting to meet him for the first time that night, I was finally able to put a face to the conversation we'd had via messenger. His genuine smile, empathetic way, and desire to please cried out to me. I could feel his hurt, his pain. I knew him through the community. He said he would be at his car for the next ten minutes and asked if I wanted a ride from the Imperial, which wasn't in the best neighborhood; Lindon Street was only a block up from where street people roamed. My friends were MIA and weren't returning my messages. I took him up on the offer and humbly agreed to a rope introduction with him at the next event. He reminded me that consent was a must, and he would ask, but it was ultimately up to me to stop and to say no. I grew nervous at this, not knowing what to expect, but I agreed and said my goodbyes after we'd talked for over an hour about life, and about how I was supposed to meet someone that night …

After several weeks, the time came when the event was happening. He picked me up and we chatted about life and what tonight would bring.

He mentioned his wife and play partner*. They were different women as this was common in the community. Fetish* isn't always about sex; it's about different sensations that turn you on. He then explained that there are different stages in bondage*, and each one was more intimate than the one before it. Full-on suspension* is more of an art form, but still a fetish. He told me that we were going to a house, and not just any house—it was a house designed for fetish play. He wouldn't say much else except that he would take me on a tour once we got there. I nodded in anxious excitement.

As we approached the house, to my surprise, it looked normal. We talked about the house and the owners. He wanted to make sure that I was feeling comfortable. The only thing was that I had nerves. Still, I was excited to explore, a beaming smile on my face. We were the first to arrive so we could see all the rooms and meet and greet the owners. They themselves used the rooms as they were kinksters*

as well. Neil led me into the kitchen, letting me know that the food
and drinks were complimentary, and that the ten-dollar cover would
suffice. They put out a spread of finger foods: a veggie tray, fruit,
cheese and crackers, and mini sandwiches topped it off; everything
was spread around the circular lime green table pushed up against
the wall. Further inside was the lounge area for socializing. It was
filled with couches and games. A movie was playing to create static
noise and comfort. This was where I met, "Cindy," the owner. She
was dressed normally, comfortably. I introduced myself and said it
was my first time here. She joked about taking my k-card (kinkster
card). I laughed. I really wanted to know how she had gotten started
running the house. She told me what her life had been like, being
into fetish, and how she had wanted her own play house. From there,
she imagined others wanting this very same thing so she decided
to share her space from time to time. Eventually, she expanded the
rooms and different areas for more types of fetish play. She urged
me to go see for myself.

I pressed Neil on exploring the rest of the house. The upstairs
had three rooms, one that belonged to the owners and was out of
bounds, and the others for aftercare*. They were for people to chill,
cuddle, debrief, rest, and clean up after playing. The room was well
stocked with cleaners, lube, condoms, towels, and lots of pillows
on a queen-size bed, which, when combined with the dim lighting,
looked very inviting. Downstairs there were five rooms. The first
one had bunk beds with kid games and books, stuffed animals, and
adult diapers, if needed, along with costumes. I was well aware that
some people fantasized about these things, but never really fully
knew that these types of rooms existed. This room was probably for
DDLG* (Daddy Dom/ Little Girl) play, for two consenting adults.
I felt awkward as I had no desire for such a scene. The next room
was bigger and had a changing table in it as well. Knowing what
it was for, but wanting confirmation, I looked at Neil, who simply
nodded. My facial expression was one of disbelief. Yes, infant play
or baby play (or ABDL*), again, for consenting adults. Underneath

the changing table were diapers, baby power, baby oil, and other essential care needs. There were even baby bottles drying on a rack by the sink. Neil pointed upward so I would notice the hooks. Rigging hooks. At least I knew what those were for. Neil told me this would be the room that we would use. He must have noticed that I was a bit nervous and that I didn't know what to do so he suggested dropping off his luggage of goodies and seeing more of the house.

The next room was filled with spank tables, toys, whips, and gadgets of all kinds. The only question I had was, "What is the rubber ducky for?" He smiled. (I still want to know what exactly that rubber ducky was for.) Knowing very well what to do in this room, I looked up to see more hooks and a cage. Play time had a new meaning in this house and I loved it. Wide-eyed, I moved forward, realizing there was another room inside this room. I opened the door to a fully decorated doctor's examination room, complete with props, coats, hats, masks, tools, bandages, and machines. The room even had a wash station for sterilizing, a needle drip, posters of the male and female reproductive systems, and two fully-functioning exam beds. In heaven, I stopped in awe of this room; when I was a little girl, I would play doctor with my friends, examining their bodies and spanking them to "find out their fat percentage." And don't get me started on playing secretary for chocolate bars.

Neil smiled as he saw my enthusiasm for this room and said I could come back here during the night as long as it wasn't occupied. There were strict rules and guidelines to follow, and the heads of the house would make sure that they were followed. If the curtain was closed, no one was to enter; likewise, a closed door meant no one enters. If it was open, you still had to ask permission to enter, even if you were trying to get into the other room inside that one. Everyone was very considerate of everyone's space, needs, and wants. Verbal consent was always upheld and everyone who had been there before knew so. Neil wanted to show me something that was hidden inside that room. He said, "If you like this room, you will love this." Looking at a small, boxed motor with a metal prong on it, I smiled, my mouth open in excitement. I had never seen one in person before, and now I would be seeing this multi-speed automatic sex machine in action, complete with unisex attachments. I could feel my blood rushing faster. I wanted to play**. He suggested asking the owner before using it as it wasn't usually available. He told me that the last time he had seen this in use, there was a line of ten people waiting to be penetrated. I told myself to focus and move on to the next room before my imagination got off track.

This room was different; cold, open-spaced. Chains, holsters, and hooks hung from the ceiling. I saw a St. Andrew's cross* against the far wall and knew instantly that this was the torture room. In this area, there was enough space for massive whips and floggers* to be used to their full extent on the individuals at hand. We passed an open metal frame filled with hooks of all angles and that was when I started fantasizing: a tied damsel in distress with a ball gag in her mouth, a black tie around her eyes, and rope tying her hair up so her head could be held straight for pleasure after being released from the gag. Her arms and legs would be tied to each post without damaging her fair skin and blonde hair. Her legs would be spread wide for her dominant partner to take her at will and fill her up as he pleased.

Neil saw me staring off into space and snapped his fingers in my face after I didn't respond to him calling me in to the next room. I shifted focus and the damsel in distress and her capturer faded away. We were still in the same room, but there was a door. Neil opened it and told me to have a look. I could feel the cold, crisp air coming from the dark room; stepping forward, I saw concrete and a wooden bench. He asked if I wanted to have the full experience. I asked what it was, and he closed the door and put the wooden 2x4 across the door. I quickly turned around and saw him waving so I played along by pounding on the door, smiling and pressing my hot hands on the tinted glass, pretending I was in pain. Moments went by and then I got a slight nervous reaction from the idea of being trapped. I heard banging, and then the heavy wood and bare metal door swung open to Neil in the doorway. He was smiling. I quickly jumped out, realizing that wasn't my jam, either. I shook my body to get rid of the chill that had come slightly over me from being in the dungeon. He asked if I was ok so I told him how cold it was in that room.

I started to warm up when he suggested we go get our shoes for outside. I looked at him wearily. He said, "The tour still isn't over." I replied with a wide-eyed, "There's more?" and grinned slightly. I quickly grabbed my jacket and shoes so I could join him. We went into the backyard where two large outdoor metal sheds stood. Opening the door to the first one, I instantly got hit by a slight, warm mist. The room was lined with candles, and the center piece was a large hot tub. I started jumping up and down like a little schoolgirl. I wanted to go in, but I knew if I did, I wouldn't come out. I examined the room a little more, looking at the care packages of lube, condoms, and other essentials that were placed in every room. This room had a radio as well, for some easy listening, if you so chose. I resisted the urge to hop in and moved to the next room, which was nothing like the sensual setting of the hot tub; this room was well lit and spacious. It was demo night for ropes and whips. There were two whippers showing off their skills to the max. This took me to a whole other level, as the whips alone were 9 to 12 feet in length; they were leather, and they made that sexy snap sound that crackles in your ears. I hadn't realized how loud it was when actually executed. I was impressed when a person stepped up to be whipped. I couldn't watch as social influence sprung up into my head, images of wrongful punishment and slavery. To my surprise, I had to leave the room at that point, and Neil realized this, too. He apologized and we went back into the house to start his demo as more and more people were showing up to explore. This place was different; people didn't dress to impress. They dressed in their street clothes, and once in the zone, they stripped down. I was used to people at Sinner's, dressing up as if it were a fashion show. (Yes, dressing up is part of the kinky way of life if it suits you.)

We returned to the room with the hooks on the ceiling and the baby changing table. He wanted to introduce me to rope before it got too busy, and then he planned on surprising me with some other gadgets he'd brought. Curiosity took hold and I didn't ask, but I acknowledged his statement. He proceeded to explain the stages of rope, and how the bottom* has to surrender to the top rigger*, and just let the sensation take over. Getting tied up is part one. He tied me up all while moving me ever so gently. I closed my eyes to better my experience, and he shut the door. The gestures and movements were only for us to experience, as they could bring up emotions and sensations that were intimate in nature. He announced every move before he did it and asked me how I was every now and then to make me feel comfortable. He would also let me know if and when he was getting close to my private areas so as not to startle me or cross a line. I told him it was all fine as long as he didn't linger. I felt the rope slither across my skin as if it were alive, slow to start then a fast, slight burning sensation from the friction. The zipping sound of the rope across my front to down in between my thighs and back up again was soothing. He would gently place the rope as if I were hot lava and he didn't want to burn himself. He was kind and gentle, swaying me with the rope as he pulled, tugged, and repositioned my body into a more restrictive pose. Suddenly, while mesmerized by the sounds and thrills, I felt my arms being held down by the sheer strength of the rope. Getting my feet tied together was another sensation altogether as some areas were more sensitive to touch than others. I could see now how this was a powerful draw for many. After he finished, he asked if I wanted to be suspended. I thought I would rather learn the next stage of rope instead, so he agreed. I opened my eyes, and he took a picture for me of my back, with a nicely designed rope flower to symbolize my beauty. I flushed at this kind gesture.

He untied me as I was dazed and told me that the next stage involved a different kind of rope, one that was harsher, coarser. He turned off the lights and instructed me to kneel on the floor. He said this would be a more sensual experience because he would be close to my back and moving his body in sync with mine. When I kneeled,

I could then feel what he meant. He reminded me that I should let him know if anything made me uncomfortable and that he would ask for permission as we went.

Not knowing what to expect, me on the ground with him kneeling behind me, I closed my eyes. He brushed the rope against me, moving it across my body and down my exposed back. I'd taken off my shirt in the previous scene. The rope felt brittle and raw across my chest and along my back. He used it to move me, sway me, and release me down only to snap me back again. I soon realized how sexual it was, more so than the last session. My heart was racing, and I could feel his heart as well. We were in sync, his hot breath pressed against my neck. He had me smell the rope, and it hit me that I wasn't in fact turned on by the rope at all, but by the process of surrender it took in order to play. I had to trust him, move with him; I loved how he controlled my movements as I went with every motion. He asked to kiss my neck. I replied with a simple nod. He kissed my neck and my back while he teased my body with the rope and its sharp tingling sensation.

He wanted more and asked to kiss me. I stopped and thought about everything and replied with a simple, "No, thank you." He agreed to respect my boundary and proceeded to preserve my comfort zone. Moments later, he asked if we wanted to push forward; I asked for the full details of that venture. He explained how it can be really intense, and that it was more sexual because I would be lying down with him on top of me, tying and playing. I had had enough; the smell of the brittle rope didn't turn me on like I thought it would. Neil respected my wishes and thanked me for trusting him to get to this point. I was amazed that he was such a gentleman, and I thanked him as well. We turned on the lights, and I put my shirt back on. He asked if he could flog me. I smirked and asked, "How big is it?" He laughed and pulled out a big one, soft and ready to use. I bent over the changing table, trying not to think about its use. He asked if I was ready. I laughed and said, "I was born ready." He loved my sense of humor and how easygoing I was. He proceeded to flog me in a gentle, sexual way, making figure eights on my ass and lower back. I thought to myself, *Wow, this is nice.* I thought it might hurt, but it was gentle and sweet. He told me that you have to know how to use a flogger the right way to make it feel this good. I said, "Well, you make it feel great." We both laughed. He said, "You're making this hard." "What am I making hard?" I smirked. He sighed and breathed out the sexual frustration I had whipped up. I stood and told him thank you. When we opened the door, a lot more people poured in. Neil was ready for the demos with everyone; he'd saved the special surprise for me.

He rounded up a few people; he would be using the same room. He pulled out his wand*, which I had never seen before, and said, "Let's learn about electrical play*," with a grin. I was shocked and excited by all the attachments he pulled out to demo. He said the louder it is, the less sensation it will have; quieter meant more zap or kick. There was an attachment for your head that produced a tingling sensation; another that made chills move through your body; yet another that felt as if a knife were cutting into your skin. One girl really enjoyed that attachment. Her and her boyfriend played in front of us. He glided it along her big, busty breasts. I creeped on every sensation and movement. After seeing all the attachments and learning about the wand itself, I was in awe at how much you could do with it.

Before everyone decided it was time to leave, he had one more demo to do. I looked over at him. He said that I would love this one. Fire play* was up next. We did it on my arms, legs, back, and bare chest. It was cool and didn't feel like it was fire since he safely swept it away after a moment's time. He also had a fire extinguisher on hand. The experience sent me back to my youth, a time when I was a little fire starter, always zapping my zippo on my leg and playing with it between my fingers for a nice little fix. Now that I knew how it felt, I would make sure and only play with someone who had been doing it for a while so I could fully trust them with lighting my body on fire. The cool blue flame was exciting to watch. After he was finished, we opened the door up to sounds of sighs, wails, moans, spanking, and pounding. The house was in full swing, and I couldn't wait to bring someone here next time.

I peeked outside the door to see a loud bottom getting spanked so hard that her ass was starting to become blue, and veins were starting to show on her plump butt. Neil said he had another girlfriend there who was from the States and wanted to get tied up. She was good with me watching. He tied her up quickly, sweat dripping down his face. He told her to brace herself as she was getting suspended. He held her legs to help her into position. She almost hit me in the face in the process. The room was small but doable, and usually there would be no one else in the room except the roper and ropee. She wasn't supposed to be talking to anyone except Neil so I decided to leave and take a peek around while I waited for them to finish. He was a master at Shibari*.

Moving my way through the people, I could see that all the other rooms were closed off and occupied, even the bunk beds with the kid toys. I wanted to watch but wasn't allowed. I wound my way upstairs to the lounge area where about eight people were sitting. They instantly welcomed me into the conversation.

I played Gameboy with one before asking some questions about how bottoms* and tops* work; would the top be more dominating or giving? And the bottom submissive? Or just enduring it? They went on to answer that Doms* are respectful, giving tops, while subs* are trusting bottoms who surrender themselves. I asked if they ever switched*, and they laughed and said they tried once and never again. They had felt out of place and uncomfortable switching roles. They even considered if they disliked it because it was out of their comfort zone, but nope, it just wasn't their thing. They had been partners in kink** for a little while, and both had other partners that they also loved. I was surprised at how common this was, to have a partner only for spanking, no sexual stuff, just kink.

They asked me if I was a top or a bottom. I said I had no idea as I was new to this and hadn't explored much up to this point. I did know that I liked both but was much more submissive than dominating in nature. Since it was getting late, Neil came back upstairs. He had agreed to drive me home early so I could get up for work the next day. I was working the weekend and needed some well-deserved sleep. Along the way, he asked me how my experience was and if I would go back, but I suspect he knew I would when the time came. I told him that it wasn't the rope that turned my sexual vixen on after all; it was the dominating nature or motion and movements that did.

## The Lessons

Going to a place with a guy you've only met once isn't the best idea; mind you, he was the best person to go with at this point in my life, and such a kind soul as well.

Quick tip: Get the address and text it to your friend so they know your location. Also tell them what time you will be home. This way you know others have your back if anything goes wrong.

Only after exploring will you truly know what you like and don't like. I thought I was into rope play, when in fact, I was more into the dominating nature of a masculine essence controlling me and moving me with deliberateness. This made it so I could surrender into my feminine essence.

Going to a play party, not just for play, but for meeting, greeting, and asking questions, is a big plus. The room upstairs was perfect for meeting people and learning about what goes on in their minds and in the community in general. If you don't ask, you won't know. Put yourself out there in order to explore. Hint: There are munches*, which are gatherings for BDSM* like-minded people to meet and greet.

Always trust your intuition and your boundaries* as there lies your integrity. I made sure not to traverse my comfort zone by speaking up. No one can read your mind so make sure you speak up for yourself. Maybe create a safe word** from the start!

Tip: Have a verbal and non-verbal cue to stop. Discuss before your scene.

Just because it doesn't rock your boat doesn't mean it won't for someone else. Everyone has their own unique inner fantasy; don't judge when it isn't the same as yours. Stay curious and ask questions if you can ... you never know what you may be able to learn about and possibly explore ...

Needless to say, sometimes the universe, or whatever, makes sure you meet or don't meet the right people for your future ...

Lastly, if you want to use a room, make sure you get there early or else you might never get in. (I'm still waiting to use that doctor's room.)

# Glossary

*ABDL*: Adult baby diaper lovers. As the name implies, ABDL involves role playing while wearing diapers, changing out of them, and so on. Fun fact—ABDL has been around a while. There is even a scholarly paper by Tuchman and Lachman, dating back to 1964.

*Aftercare*: After a scene—yes, you guessed it—you care for each other (usually, the sub needs extra care). This can look like going into a separate room to check-in and cuddle, for possibly easing back into a comfy headspace to finish your scene with more even care and togetherness. Or it can mean asking for certain things or certain kinds of support. Aftercare is important because lots of chemicals release when you are highly stimulated, which in turn can cause a down/deplete later on, a.k.a. a "con drop." Things that help include rehydration/replenishment; caring for aches, pains, or marks/bruises; taking a tiny nap; check-ins/talking; and/or maybe a massage.

*BDSM*: Bondage, discipline, dominance and submission, sadomasochism. BDSM is the term used for certain kinds of erotic play between consenting adults. Bondage is described below. Discipline is a type a punishment that is done through rule breaking or for fun. Dominance and submission are described below, as well as bottom and top. The sadomasochism* element of BDSM represents the act of deriving pleasure by giving or receiving pain, torture, or humiliation.

*Bondage*: In BDSM subculture, bondage is the practice of tying, binding, or restraining someone consensually.

*Bottom*: This term is used to refer to a certain sexual or psychological preference for the role of the submissive or passive. This does not necessarily mean the person is sexually on the bottom.

*Boundaries*: Where you end and the other begins; what you're ok and nor ok with.

*DDLG or Daddy Dom/Little Girl Play*: This kind of play involves consenting adults who may or may not dress up. They satisfy each other's needs by giving/getting the care and attention they need/crave. Dom daddies exert positive masculinity (and mommies exert a nurturing femininity). A "little" acts as if they are a child.

*Dom*: Persons who take a "dominant" role are Doms (male) or Dommes (female).

*Edgeplay or Edging*: In BDSM, edgeplay or edging means riding the edge. However, edgeplay focuses on the psychological mindfuck and on expanding what you think you can handle, while edging focuses on riding the edge of an orgasm. You can do this with breathing, being present, slowing down, or taking breaks. Edging can prolong your orgasm, produce a more powerful orgasm, or help you enjoy the journey and sensation of being in the moment.

*Electrical Play*: This type of play usually involves a wand (see glossary), with attachments that can be adjusted according to your desired strength. The wand is a medical device from the Victorian era that is now used as a sex toy, and/or for edgeplay* or edging* and stimulation.

*Fetish*: To have a fetish is to enjoy a nonsexual object or body part sexually. Common fetishes include feet and shoes, leather, or rubber.

*Fire Play*: Here, alcohol was set on fire on the skin. This BDSM practice is exactly what the name implies—playing with fire in a safe manner. Every time I have had friends do fire play, safety measures—such as a fire extinguisher—were always present.

*Flogger*: A flogger is a BDSM/kink toy that is used to "flog" someone. Flogging involves technique and the range of sensation can go from light and sensual to thudding or stinging, depending on what the players desire and discussed beforehand. In a non-BDSM context, you can also see floggers used for horses. They are made out of leather with a handle at one end.

*Kinksters*: People who enjoy kinky things or kinks.

*Munches*: These are social gatherings for BDSM, Kink, or Lifestyle people to gather under relaxed settings. They usually happen at a restaurant, bar, lunch spot, or over coffee. The goal is to find like-minded people and connect to the community.

*Play Partner*: A play partner is someone who may or may not be a person's primary partner. A play partner is someone you scene or play out a fetish with. The scene does not usually include penetration but can if discussed beforehand and consent is given.

*Rigger*: A riggers ties (a) person(s) up in a sexual kink/BDSM context. The rigging can vary from ceiling hooks to crosses. This player is very aware and focused on the play partner that they are tying. They are also very skilled and will have discussed safety, safe words, and the play partner's needs with the play partner. This knowledge will allow them to focus on the tension of the whole experience as well as on expressing their mastery and on recognizing if something isn't working.

*Scene*: A time when a BDSM/kink/lifestyle activity occurs; includes different types of play that are discussed beforehand.

*Shibari*: Ancient Japanese rope play, bondage.

*St. Andrew's Cross*: This type of cross is shaped like an "X." These types of crosses allow for tying, flogging, playing, blindfolding, or whatever the sub/Dom wants to play around with. A St. Andrew's cross is usually leather bound with tie-down rings on four or more points. Its name refers to a story in which Saint Andrew was said to have been martyred by crucifixion.

*Sub*: Persons who take the subordinate position are called "submissive" or "subs" (male or female).

*Suspension*: Suspension occurs when you're tied up and off the ground, suspended in air with rope.

*Switch*: A switch goes back and forth between two preferences, usually bottom and top and depending on the scene.

*Top*: This term is used to refer to a certain sexual or psychological preference for the role of the dominant or active partner when playing. This does not necessarily mean the person is sexually on top.

*Wand a.k.a. the violet wand*: This device uses an Oudin coil to apply low-current, high-voltage electricity to the body. The wand has medical benefits and is also used in sadomasochistic* sex play.

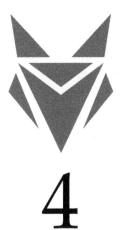

# 4

# NYE 14-HOUR SEX SHOW

~He was taller than me, a blond ginger; the kind that would confuse you and make you laugh. He was kind, gentle, and lovable. Without a doubt, he knew all this about himself. His grace shined and his charm filled the room. It was hard to know if he was flirting with only you or with everyone. He was young, strong, and very fit. He wanted a change in scenery. His light piercing-blue eyes told a story I knew too well, one of trouble and pain, but he hid it well within his solidly built walls. He made sure not to show too much or bare too much, so he could decide to have the glass half full or half empty, to eat a piece of cake or eat the whole thing as well, to have one foot in and the other out. He always needed to have an escape, to not be seen as he didn't see himself yet.~

The pre-party was in full swing! I was at a different party than the one he was at. Secretly piling in the bathroom, I dipped my finger in molly and shoved it up my friend's ass as he bent over the toilet in a downtown penthouse; my other friend tugged on his balls with a moan. He loved it and wanted more. After round two, he turned around, whipped out his dick and told me to do a line on it.

Mysteriously creeping out from the bathroom, we found five others drinking, swaying and ready as we cheered once more to what the night had in store. This was only the start … the rest of the night was ahead of us …

It had started like any other night, except tonight was NYE. After dancing up a storm, kissing everyone at the stroke of midnight, and enjoying my girlfriend's tongue down my throat, it was time for the next party. My party, and my man's at the time, was ending at the same time, and nothing and everything was met. Inevitably, NYE was a hit by 1:00 am, and I started walking towards *him* on a night I knew I would never forget. This guy was pursuing me, and I was pursuing him …

We kept texting as I kept walking towards the party he was at. Something wasn't right. I looked up to see the hotel my boy was partying at. Then I saw him—he was holding another girl; she was mesmerized by him, looking up at his 6'1" blond-redhead, blue-eyed gorgeousness. She was in his arms, wrapped in his jacket.

Shocked, I went up to him, shouting, *What the Fuck?!* in my head. I gave him a *WTF?!* look of disapproval. He turned and looked at me in complete shock—a blank, pale, big-eyed, *I'm caught* look. I instantly understood and said hi to her. "I'm Z." She said, "Hi, I'm Amanda." In my head, her name was *skank*. She gave my "date" a what-the-fuck look with her eyes.

He told me to wait while he made his goodbye rounds. He said goodbye to his friends and was coming my way when SHE ran into his arms; he grabbed her—no question, no hesitation, not even a flinch. I thought, *Do I leave, or do I stay?* I tried to be logical, reasonable, while I contemplated how to deal with this situation. I should have left, but I didn't. I should have told him it wasn't cool, but I didn't. The happy pills I'd had earlier in the night made it even more difficult to decide. I stared at my shadow. I liked him, and I knew this situation wouldn't keep me from someone I enjoyed.

When I looked back up, they were kissing, and I just sank. My stomach turned, and I was in shock once again. I should have reacted, and in that moment, I should have just left. Hans, the guy from the bathroom, asked me what was up. He was bouncing from side to side, his eye twitching every so often, all hyped up on drugs, drinking, and more. Persistent, Hans said he would treat me right and give me the attention I deserved if we left. He nodded over at my date and said screw him.

Again, I analyzed the situation; I wanted to give my date the benefit of the doubt and let him tell me his story. He walked over as I gazed disappointedly in his direction. My eyes reflected the hurt I felt, and I didn't say anything for a bit. While we walked, I was trying to find how to get to DT Core from the hotel. I told myself our next destination was going to be fabulous as I knew that my emotions wouldn't fully show because the happy pills were masking them. I was also hiding my emotions, swallowing them down. I then asked who she was. He paused and said, "No one. Just a girl I met at the party, but I left with you." He didn't look at me. He must have known that answer wouldn't suffice because it didn't explain why they had been making out like love bugs, bringing in the New Year all by themselves.

When we arrived at our destination through the back entrance, we undressed, stuffed our belongings into lockers, and set sail into the club at once. As he grabbed my arm and pushed me to the dance floor, I gestured *one sec* with my finger and rushed to the bathroom to fix my unruly hair and check my makeup; surprisingly, it was flawless, my big fake lashes batting away. I reached into my bag and made my night a little more pleasurable by pressing down the other half of the molly I'd had, all the while making sure I had a full one for Dave, my date. As we headed out from the unisex washroom to the dance floor, I knew when the music poured into my ears that this would be a fun night. He motioned me for a drink, after which I shook the pill free for him. We drank and looked around the club to take in the scene. I had no expectations; I just wanted to let my friend molly take me through the night.

The room next to the bar was the show room, where plexiglass allowed you to show off like exhibitionists* by doing a scene** together for spectators to watch. After grabbing his hand and pulling him onto the platform, I pulled his pants down, seducing him with my eyes as I slithered my way down to his big, thick cock. I was drooling for its taste and its erection. He grabbed the back of my head to help motion me in on him, and away I went, worshiping his cock as if it were sacred and rare. I licked his veins, feeling them swell up to the tip of his cock. I licked his dick from tip down to his smooth scrotum and back, bringing my hands into play. As I slurped, I could feel him shaking his leg; he pulled me up and whispered that he couldn't do it here anymore because the four men masturbating to our show were throwing him off his game. I turned around and smiled as he pulled his pants up and we made our way off the platform. Our audience had been giving us praise, commenting about how hot we were. If I'd had a mirror, I could've watched us. This club was a sex-positive* SOP* club, and boy, was it ever!

Pushing forward to the next new scene, I saw four curtains and opened one up. There were individual playrooms that only fit one to two people max. Three were already in use, so we took the last one. Getting high on his taste and sweat, I eagerly pushed him in and started kissing him passionately. He stopped to look around the room, then smiled as he closed the curtain so his half-naked ass wasn't hanging out. I grabbed him closer to me and pushed his pants down. In the distance, he sneaked a peek at my friend Ryder, who hooted, "Ooh, you love birds." I smiled as Dave kissed me, only momentarily wondering why he had ignored Ryder's teasing, but thought nothing more of it at the time. Sex and lust ruled me that night. I started giving him a hand job until he couldn't handle it anymore; after feeling how wet I was, he spun me around and pressed me up against the wall, kissing the backside of my neck before pushing his thick, luscious dick fully inside me, sliding it around my wet vagina. He glided in and out, thrusting hard, his hot breath against the back of my neck. He wrapped his arms around my front for easy access to my perky boobs and held me close.

Following his lead, I grabbed the wall in front of me for leverage and pounded back into him, in sync with his movements. Dripping with sweat, I turned around, wanting to see and taste him. I went down and licked, fondled, and teased away again. Dave didn't like it all that much or maybe it was that he just wanted in me again; either way, he pulled me back up and sat on the bench so I could sit on top of him and feel every inch of him inside of me. I moved slightly, playing with his dick inside of me—pulsing, moving, tensing. He kept asking me, in a mind-blown kind of way, how I was doing this and how it felt so good. I would only reply with a smile and keep playing.

Breathless, we looked at each other and smiled. I asked him if he had kissed her at midnight. He said no, but I could feel that he was being off. I sensed a lie, but at this point, I didn't want to deal with it, especially since he'd said earlier, "I'm leaving with you." I wanted to believe him so the next thing he said eased my misgivings; he told me he'd been waiting for me. We smiled and I said, "Well, let's have our own countdown, naked, me on top of you and you inside me." So we started counting down from five together as the music blared, our only light coming from the flickering, staggered lights of the dance floor. One on one, we made our memory of the night, still plugged into each other, kissing passionately.

The moment passed and our mood changed; we still wanted to dance the night away, so we got dressed and made our way to the dance floor. Engulfing ourselves in the musical beats of DJSPANK, doing it up right for those left at 5:00 am, we knew we wanted to sway while vibrational beats penetrated our bodies. She put on "Faded" by ZHU and we moved through the dance floor, half naked and embracing the rhythmic flow of our bodies. Dave was clearly high; he loved me feeling his every move. He was in awe, closing his eyes and raising his arms to the sensational tingling feelings that arose. Ryder was looking at Dave in his underwear, speechless at his six-pack, 6'1" model body. Dave had no idea—not yet anyway. I winked at Scott passing by, acknowledging his smirk. I knew his intentions, as Scott was bi and liked what he saw.

Edging over to another playroom, I cat-walked in, leading Dave by the hand. We nudged our way to the very back room, equipped with a dungeon master*, sex swing, sitting bench, spank tables, and a swinging red-leather bed that caught my eye. I smiled at him as we wiped the sex swing clean. He pushed me onto it; it swung back and forth, mounted from the ceiling by heavy-duty chain-link, good for grabbing on to. I helped him take my bottoms off and we were once more putting on a show. But this time my friend Hans was there, playing with himself and asking me if he could tap in and have a taste. My date looked up and said, "He has no filter." I laughed and replied, "You just found that out?"

Dave wanted more and I tried to help him by repositioning myself, for my pleasure, but the swing wasn't the thing; we made it work anyway as he was good at what he did down there. Moaning and clutching the chain, I grabbed Dave's hair and arched my back while curling my toes and giving myself up to such sexual pleasure. I let go and embraced satisfaction. I wanted more; I whispered in his ear, "Stick it in me." He didn't hesitate and pulled his underwear down, but again the swing wasn't working for our play so we stopped and cleaned up before moving on to more solid ground. We wanted to have full control over the situation. As we were leaving, Hans clapped and said, "Holy fuck, thank you, can I have a turn?" He had a big drunk grin on his face, and he licked his lips as if I were an appetizer. I replied, "No, thank you." After he'd asked me earlier that night if he could eat my pussy and taste my nectar on the way to Hotel Ontario, it was easy to say no a second time.

Dave and I moved around, tumbling as we went. My legs were

trembling with pleasure and his legs were getting sore as well. We knew there was more night to go for us since we always had our own after-party—only for us. We progressed to the bathroom to have some more fun and for me to slurp my way to his pounding. We came out the other side, parched and ready for our round at home ...

Our party consisted of music, dancing, and nonstop, all-night sex until we were too tired to keep going or the sun told us it was time to take a nap. Either way, we always made the best of a situation. Resting, touching, sexing till we were famished and unable to move ...

## The Lessons

First off, when or if you find out your guy is with another girl and starts making out with her in front of you, hold your ground and know your worth!

That is a big indicator of a lack of respect, a lack of trust, and a lack of boundaries** on both sides. He truly didn't know his own boundaries either, and he didn't even know what to say to the other girl. He could have spoken up, and I could have said, "Hey, I'm his gf," as well—just to see how that would play out. It would have been funny, but only at the time; later though, I would have felt crappy for ruining that girl's night. Leading someone on when you have someone already, without saying anything to either girl, is just a sneaky way of fooling around, and people get hurt in the process. Trust me, we all find out. The truth eventually comes out.

You must express your own boundaries within a relationship openly. The sooner, the better. As soon as you know you're not the right match for each other, the less time you waste and the less room for hurt. If you find out you're a solid match, then great! More room for fun and adventures together. But remember—there are different types of boundaries: rigid, which are *heck noes*; or porous, ones that you'd rather not have crossed but let others cross them anyway, without repercussion. Healthy is what we aim for. Healthy boundaries work when things happen maybe once, and there are consequences; you know how to say no and yes equally and stand for your values. Boundaries change and flow over time. Do you still have the same boundaries you had five years ago or even a year ago? I would assume not. We change, our values change, and so do our boundaries. It's what makes us (and others) understand what's ok and what's not ok.

Brushing things off can trigger your fight, flight, or freeze response*, which is a survival mechanism that sometimes helps and sometimes doesn't. That night, I didn't handle things properly and didn't openly express how disrespectful his behavior was or how truly hurt I was that night. I brushed it off, and every time he got hit on by another girl or he would hit on another girl, I would walk away from the situation, not knowing to how to deal with it. In some situations, this led to a passive-aggressive attitude and me feeling like I couldn't express myself fully with him. This in turn caused us to grow apart, among other things, down the road.

Years later, we are still friends and happy ones at that. Allowing space between us, as well as time and healing, helped us grow into a better way of being, and to this day, I wouldn't date him, but he sure is a lot of fun!

## Glossary

*Dungeon Master a.k.a. Dungeon Monitor*: a person who monitors the play space. To make sure consent is followed, there are safe sex practices, as well as a designated person to come to if there is an issue. Dungeon masters (or monitors) are clearly indicated, usually by tag, introduction, or uniform.

*Exhibitionist*: An exhibitionist likes putting on a show for others, and they get aroused by doing so. Usually, exhibitionism is consensual, and it is often associated with voyeurism, which occurs when someone becomes aroused by watching others put on a show. Voyeurism is also usually consensual.

*Fight, Flight, or Freeze Response*: When your lovely body activates its fight, flight, or freeze response, it is attempting to protect you from danger. This survival mechanism prompts you to either escape, fight for your life, or freeze so as to be ignored or not "seen." In BDSM play, this response can either help you or hold you back. There is another option referred to as "fawn," in which a sub basically agrees to whatever the Dom decrees in order to save themselves.

*Sex-Positive*: Normalizing sexuality for pleasure as a consent culture.

*SOP*: Sex on the premises.

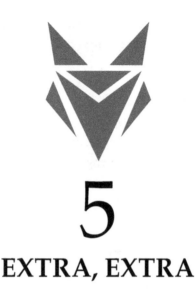

# 5

## EXTRA, EXTRA

~He was only a little taller than me, with dark hair and eyes to match. With one glance in each other's direction, we knew, without a doubt, how the night would go. His grace and presence were mysteriously deceiving, and his smile gave off an interested and interesting allure. He would constantly joke around and call me his "set wife number four"; he'd been doing set work for a while now. He showed me the tips and tricks of film: always pay attention; complain about everything except your boredom; hide among the crowd and never stand out except when told; never engage the actors unless approached, and don't talk on set or else you will get yelled at, or worse, not called back. You basically rush there for your call time to sit and wait on set. Wardrobe, hair, and makeup was a line-up process. After signing in and filling out paperwork, we started sneaking out outside since it was spring, and the weather was clear. His flask was full; it tasted like apple cider. Luke and I knew instantly our hidden game, one that would stay hidden for now.~

*C*all time was 18:00 with an unknown end. Pay was minimal, and they had to pay you for four hours by law. The scene was a grand ball. Luckily, I was pre-fitted for this G-rated scene. Looking around at the others, I saw what they considered G-rated, and I was extremely amused at their interpretation: short, see-through cocktail dresses. One wore fake diamonds that covered her privates. I couldn't hold in my laughter at that point.

I was amused and ready for shooting to begin. Since it was past my bedtime, I started writing a little into the book I was working on—yes, this one. He sat next to me as we joked about how "hideous" I looked while all clean and sparkly. I wanted to choke him with his maroon business tie; the tie itself was practically taunting me to do so. As we got called into set, I put my book away. We continued hazing each other and trying to make the other slip up. Then we were sent back into holding. Since everyone else was sleeping, I rested my eyes until we were called again.

My rest was disrupted by a paper hitting my head. I opened my eyes to see everyone lined up to leave and Luke laughing. I gathered my black heels in my hand and headed to the door, trying to add body back to my hair by pushing it up. While we lined up like we were getting picked for teams, I quietly joined in. One by one, everyone got paired off by the AD (Assistant Director).

Luke and I were paired together as if we already were together, after the AD joked that we matched on purpose. We looked at each other; neither of us had realized that we were color-coordinated. Before long, we knew what the other was thinking. His mind was as dirty as mine. We sat together, worked together, and had dressed to match without even realizing it. The desire was overpowering for both of us, to the extent that we could not concentrate. Our thoughts of pleasure and embracing became reality.

The extra waiting around and the secret hiding places within the building had made it even more thrilling and taboo. We had just met, but we already felt so much, and it was as if we had known for a while what was coming. We didn't fight it; we embraced all of it.

We were like lost lovers that hadn't seen one another for months or years. Our hearts beat like we'd been celibate all that time as well. Our inner beasts were itching, craving, and clawing at all the other thoughts in their way.

The room was full of directors, actors, and ADs, but none were looking our way nor were they even close to realizing what we were up to. The room was alit with chandeliers and lights lined around white, mini-tree centerpieces at every table. Pearl-white tablecloths draped down to the floor, where yet another satisfying hiding place awaited. The tables were lit up with candles and props of cocktails waiting to be sipped, and the room was lined with pillars spaced out elegantly as if in a Roman temple. I had worn my deep red, strappy dinner dress and flashy "diamond" earrings and necklace. He was in a black suit with a shirt that matched my dress. We laughed hysterically while muttering, "You've got to be kidding me," while gazing into each other's eyes. It was as if it were meant to be. We soon realized no one could see us or hear us where we were.

We found corners during the shoot and slithered away to become one for the moment. We slipped behind a pillar while Luke gently glided his hand lower and lower down my lower back, sending chills up my spine. I had to close my eyes and bite my lip. Taking my hand, he spun me until I was backed up against the pillar with him pressed against me; the cold pillar contrasted lusciously with my hot mess of a body. He slid his hand up my thigh, slowly moving it up and inward, towards my lace thong. My breathing quickened, and my heart raced. I narrowed my eyes at him as he held my hands up and away so I couldn't say no. He whispered in my ear, "I dreamt about this last night." His hot breath on my neck and ear reminded me of tea in a meadow, which made me melt as I closed my eyes to embrace the moment, no longer fighting it.

As intrigued and indulgent as I'd become, I could feel myself throbbing with each move; I wanted the teasing to stop. Frustration levels from playing around were too high. We had to go behind the next unlocked door and lock it once more.

He pushed me inside, and I turned around to him charging me, grabbing my head and engulfing my luscious mouth. He pressed me down on the desk. Fumbling and breathing heavily, he pushed himself on top of me as I undid his slick jacket bottoms and untucked his maroon shirt. Lust took over my entire body, and I let my beast run fully wild—no shame, no judgment, no agenda, only pleasure. He moved his hand from my chest to the bottom of my dress, and throwing it up, he secured my body fully on top of the table. I moaned with the satisfaction of being taken—pleased, embracing my desires, my vixen goddess, my inner wolf.

I threw my head back as he moved his carpenter's hands between my legs, pushing my lace underwear aside in eagerness. He pressed two fingers inside my wet pussy, and I bit my lip when he started quickly thrusting his fingers in and out, fast, before knowing whether or not I was ready for them yet. I grabbed his shirt and ripped off his buttons for easy access. I unbuckled his pants to greet his throbbing, eager cock, which made his pants burst open once released. I used my own juices as lube and handled his rock-hard dick. He closed his eyes and quivered in pleasure, suddenly pressing three fingers inside me, making me flinch. He moved them out and pressed his blood-infused dick against me. I could feel him slide on the juices flowing from my pussy. I wanted him and wanted him bad. I was pulsing from his dick's motions on top of my clit. He grabbed my hair and pressed me down to demonstrate that he had total control. I couldn't stop making noise after noise. He wanted me, and he took me right then and there. When his thick, rock-hard dick pressed into me, I let out a slight *ahhh* because I wanted it and it hurt, but only slightly. As much as I wanted it, I wasn't prepared for his aggressive penetration. He pounded me, held my hair down, and grabbed my ass to direct me wherever he wanted me. I couldn't help but scream with excited pleasure. He had to muffle my noise, ironically, with his tie. He wanted me to take his load in my mouth, but he blew before he could position me to take it …

I jolted and opened my eyes, breathing heavy. My vision was blurry. I realized I was still in holding as a paper ball hit me in the head. Luke was telling me, "Get up, princess." I hurried, put my book away, and grabbed my heels. All the while, I was thinking, *Did I just dream it all …*

July 25th was our sex date. On the phone, he described a luscious dream of delicious secrecy on set. We had both felt the chemistry and had both been taken aback by it, but we laughed it off as if we both knew never to cross that line. It was still fun to experience it in a dreamscape where we could both satiate our urges.

## The Lessons

So don't fall asleep writing about sex stuff on set or your head will go on a crazy ride, not that I'm complaining. Try denying having flushed cheeks to everyone around you and slowly wondering if it was even a dream or thinking about how real it was to you. Let's look at this closer, shall we? It's perfectly normal to fantasize*, dream about, think about others, but actually doing it is another thing. "Look, but don't touch" comes to mind right away unless you're single, both willing, open to it, or in a different type of relationship dynamic—with consent, of course. We both weren't at that point in the game. We both had someone we cared about, but we teased each other about it at the same time. Plus working together … Can you imagine the drama now?

Monogamish* was another possibility that showed up on the radar. Sometimes it's fun to talk with your partner about doing things with others—not necessarily engaging in them, but flirtatiously playing with the idea of it. If you haven't heard about it, there is a Ted Talk on "monogamish" available to watch on YouTube.

This one was a breather chapter, for the dreamer and creator.

Wet dreams!

# Glossary

*Fantasize*: We often dream or daydream about things we might be longing to try. The key here is that fantasizing doesn't mean you actually want the fantasy to happen; fantasizing is your mind wandering all over the place and going over taboo possibilities it wants to play out! Yes, I'm talking about sexual fantasies here. Consent is necessary when you actually do want to see a fantasy through, as well as having that good ol' boundary chat and establishing a safe word. For example, you might want to explore a sexual rape fantasy where saying no is part of the fantasy, but you will need a certain word, agreed upon ahead of time, to use if you need to call a complete stop to the situation. When does fantasy become a tad unhealthy? When it affects your daily life and you are constantly longing for what you're fantasizing about. Most fantasies are just that—fantasies

*Monogamish*: This is a great term for people who aren't quite non-monogamy nor are monogamy. They kind of dabble on the edge and play within or dip their toe in some light non-monogamy flirtatious play and toy with the idea with their whomever. This idea come around when some people come to certain events, may put on a show or tell their partner certain wild things they would like to do with others, etc. but not actually do it. However, there are different definitions of this, as well, I believe in creating a relationship based on what relationship you want to create together and not a label that defines it.

# 6

# MR. KINK

~His name was "Mr. Kink." He swayed and moved as if his body's muscles were the rhythm. His innocent blue eyes pierced everyone else unwittingly mesmerized by his perception. He sat by me and read a page of my book, after which he asked when I would be finished. My eyes gazed at his, knowing his agenda by his kind. I replied with a gentle, "Until I realize my curiosity." His eyes gleamed and told me that he could let me in. We paused when we realized we were both in the same scene—same interests and damn gleaming eyes that told another story.~

He was hot, young, blond, strong and wanted to play**. He always had a crazy mind, as one might put it. To me, he was one of the normal ones that tested the waters and embraced the unknown willingly.

We were nervous, he more so. As we sipped on the last of

our cocktails to ease our inhibitions and encourage the taboo behaviors dying to come out, he casually progressed with me up the stairs, looking around through the windows, seeing the bricks of downtown's core, sheepishly saying *You think they can see us?* with a wink.

He put on his own show and had all the gadgets to go with any fantasy. When my curiosity requested more, he insisted on showing me and on practicing. His playroom was bigger than his bedroom. His twelve disciples were, in fact, twelve butt plugs of different sizes and colors. I thought, *At least he has variety and isn't racist.* My mind ran full speed and my eyes lit up in the toy room. Among the sex toys were the spank table, ropes, swings, and movable, shaped pillows displayed with a frame. A "prep bar" and "after station" were ready; once I feasted my eyes on that, Garden of Eve popped into my head, and I realized this was his personal version of such sexual pleasures. One phrase unconsciously popped into my head after that: *What a skank!* Laughing, he realized not everyone owns theses lovely sexy things displayed like trophies hanging on the walls. Soon, my attention swayed to the center of the room, wanting to run at it full speed and swing my body with abandon around the shiny chrome fantasy. My heart skipped a beat before my mouth could even form the words "stripper pole" —where one can show off amazing wonders of all kinds. He smiled sheepishly, aware of his skill range. I beamed up at him, as if in a challenge he had to be expecting. My mind went into amazement and overload as soon as he glided his hands, then fingertips, along the pole's shaft, swinging as he knew was his calling.

"Where shall I go?" I hesitated.

"Anywhere will do ..." he excitedly directed around the room.

He wanted me to wear his favorite 20-inch dildo so he could suck me off and beg for more. I slapped him across the face with one swift motion of the giant, wiggling hard-on I had strapped onto me. He wore a black holster and garter with sheer black tights. He wore it well and knew how to move in it, as if he had done this exact thing already. His gaze lingered low, and he went on all fours before spinning around, wanting me to pound him from behind. I was nervous, what with not knowing what I was doing, and I looked around, curious and anxious for lube. He directed me to it and told me to not be gentle once I was in. I widened my eyes … unsure how to start. I lubed up. *More is better* I was told when it came to butt play. I played with his rim and pressed the schlong against his plump, perked-up, beautiful ass. He was bent down, ready to be taken.

I wanted to please him, and I could feel the heat and energy in motion between us. I started to enter him as he moaned and motioned for me to go a little deeper inside him. I was scared. This attachment was huge, and if I were him, I would be screaming. He directed me to go in and out with the tip only, and then slow, with his cues to insert more on the thrust. His panting told me he was ready for more so I started to get into it. While he was holding on to his bed, I stood, giving him thrust after thrust, the pleasure he had longed for and desired between us. *He moans so heavenly,* I thought as I questioned if I was enjoying it.

He turned to me, wanting more and showing me another toy to use, this time on his erect dick. It was a mini peg to stick into the top of his dick, he explained, as I grinned with an open mouth. He had a small grin on his face. My gaze pierced his, my mouth open, not knowing what to expect and half-thinking he was joking. As I wondered if he was serious, he handed the peg to me, ready for more pleasure. Still half inside him, he suggested we finish with what we were doing and move on to more advanced projects. He wanted me to use him, feel him, and penetrate him into cumming from the other side and longing for more. He wanted me to be his playmate, his Dominatrix*, his woman on top. He had already told people about me and how it would be hotter and more adventurous if we both put on a show together. The audience had agreed. I was nervous, knowing but not knowing what to do. This was all new to me.

As we progressed, we paused, adjusted, and he went on top, me pushing from below and him riding from above. I felt his smooth back and pulsing muscles as he deep-dived himself onto the thick, 20-inch dildo he wanted so badly. He rode better than most women, swaying his hips in rhythmic bliss. His noises aroused me. It was empowering, intoxicating; it was moving to be in this position—the position a male is usually in—taking on, thrusting, pounding, and giving it to someone. I could see how this dominant position feels from within—taking charge, being needed, wanted, and giving it to someone who begged for more. Excitement poured all through my body. His dick was becoming aroused; he apologized as if that hadn't been agreed upon. I acknowledged his apology and allowed his arousal, all while nodding for more. He moved his body more and more, snapping the dildo's holster, breaking its threads with our fierce, passionate, masculine energy. He asked to cum, out of breath ... longing and ready to explode ... swaying his hips slowly to hold back. I saw him touching himself as I penetrated him from the back, overstimulating his senses to overdrive his urge.

I kept pegging* and moving into him as his moans became more drastic, evolving into bliss-like ecstasy. The holster was coming apart little by little, and I was holding on to the dildo with my hands, keeping it straight so not to lose our ascent towards God. I was sweating, holding and pounding as he started shaking and bursting. The harness straps were beyond repair; I was holding on for dear life. It was intense, beautiful, rhythmic, and sensational. Never had I ever had an experience like this before.

I went to get a towel, slowly lifting up and rolling towards the ground since my legs were jelly from the intense workout of being the top, from experiencing the masculine drive. He was flushed and hot as hell. The bedroom was washed in a pleasant glow from the sun setting, a wistful mist of citrus. We washed up and both lay down side by side on the bed in silence, in awe about what just happened and I started laughing. Breaking the silence, he asked, "Was it as good for you as it was for me?" He chuckled and we discussed our enjoyment, our awkwardness, and our fucking epic experience.

## Mr. Kink's Experience!

"*She was kind, sexy, and hot as hell! Her curves swayed as if she knew what she was doing, and all while making my body tremble with desire. Her dark hair glistened with highlights of red in the sunlight, making her green eyes pop even more. Her smile was contagious—straight, white teeth and plump, kissable lips. Au natural and all. Her best ass-et was her fine bubble butt that was a real showstopper and her personality that took no prisoners—she was a smart one. Her fit, model 5'8" figure was dressed to impress. Her name was ... 'Vixen.'*

*I remember feeling anxious and excited in anticipation for what was to come. I'm bold and open, but as you know ... I can certainly be shy and my sub\*\* side shines through when I need to be nudged along. That was also the case here ... catching up ... warming up with you again, and then getting to an evening that I'll never forget. I remember taking the big dildo out to show you what you would be using on me ... The excitement as I held it in my hand in front of you and put it into the harness ... Slowly going down on my knees to fasten the buckles on the sides to secure it on your gorgeous frame ... Running my hand down your leg and making sure it was comfortable ... On my knees, looking up at you with anticipation ... Your big, gorgeous member now attached to you as I had always dreamed. I put my hands on each side of your waist and kissed and licked your big member. This was it ... It was really happening ... Feeling you relax into it and grab the back of my head to guide me helped as I opened my mouth ... and slowly took in the tip ... and out ... then deeper the next time ... and deeper ...*

*closing my eyes and opening them as I looked up at you and your facial expressions. I took the entire member down my throat and held it there, pulling it out and gasping ... but very much eager to please and to make sure you enjoyed every minute of it.*

*My own member now dripped from arousal. We climbed up on the bed and I bent over on all fours while you cozied up behind me. I held my breath. I was hoping you were enjoying the view and could only imagine what you were thinking as my mind was racing and I was in a state of euphoria. I could feel the head of your member kissing my spread cheeks as you eased it inside ... opening me up ... I moaned and held my breath. You were very hung, but I wanted every inch of you inside me. I slowly rocked back, taking in every inch of you again ... this time, in my other hole. It felt amazing ... You were hitting my g-spot on your first try. A natural. Well worth the wait and I loved every minute of it!*

*Feeling your hands on my hips as you dominated me was heaven. I wanted more and more. We changed positions, and this time, I rode on top of you. Cowgirl ... Rocking onto you from the top ... I controlled the pace now and worked myself again to orgasm.*

*You were such a gorgeous, natural pegger. I was beyond happy to be taken by you. The only regret was we didn't have multiple toys, ranging in size, and a much better harness ... which prevented me from really working that toy hard for you.*

*Not a day goes by that I don't think of that amazing session.*

*Thank you for pegging me.*
*Mr. Kink"*

## The Lessons

You're welcome. This is your intermission and pleasure chapter. It was consensual for all parties. My BF at the time told me it would be a great experience for you, and I was happy about his hand in it. We had had a few chats beforehand, and for that matter, we were friends who knew this was an experience that we both wanted and got huge pleasure from. Yes, I was a Dom** for an evening, and it was empowering! This isn't for everyone, however; the experience was the right fit for both sides. I lucked out with Mr. Kink. He is a femmey* that is taking her power more and more as I see him grow. Moral of this story: Don't knock it till you try it or at least have a discussion about it.

## Glossary

*Dominatrix*: A woman who takes the "dominant" role in BDSM activities. One who takes the lead.

*Pegging*: A sexual practice in which a woman performs anal sex on a man by penetrating his anus with a strap-on dildo.

*Femmey/Femme:* In this context, the male bringing out his feminine role, with more feminine aspects. Such as wearing female lingerie, wigs, being more submissive, etc. Embodies and embraces the feminine through sexy empowerment.

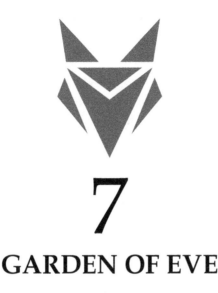

# 7

# GARDEN OF EVE

~ ... where the designation and the location has made it the legend it is today. You have to be approved in order to register and go to the club. Step one, make a profile; step two, agree to the rules; and three, wait for approval. You can get rejected. They do screen and make sure that there is a certain male-to-female ratio. You wouldn't want a sausage fest, would you? Well, this isn't that type of party. ~

*T*here are strict rules and guidelines you must sign and follow. Annual fees are paid, or guests sign in through their site; once you get a ticket, the location is revealed. Less is more when you go. Prepping for Garden of Eve in and of itself is a fun adventure. Garden of Eve is where you dress up to dress down.

As a newbie, you watch a video, sign a waiver, and are then given a grand tour by their Cupid guides. Knowing where to go and what the club has to offer, plus scouting out some epic spots for wild adventures, is definitely a must. This was my first visit to Garden of Eve and let me just say, after this night, I will definitely be going back.

Everyone who goes is dressed to the nines and gorgeous. There are buttons you can take to indicate what you want. If you're a girl looking for a girl, you wear a pink pin, so everyone knows what you're looking for, and the same thing goes for guys looking for a girl; they also wear a pink pin. Looking for a guy? Put on a blue pin. If you're a couple and just want each other, no pins necessary (I feel like an infomercial saying that one).

You walk in to be greeted at the sign-in table, where you can also find the pins. Then you wait in line to check the list and registry if you have not signed up yet. After you register, you are wrist-banded. Registration involves a bunch of paperwork and a newbie video that you are required to watch so you know what and what not to do. After that, there are lockers to lock up your clothes and get your *sexy on*; bring a lock or you'll be purchasing one.

You instantly feel welcomed and comfortable as others start chatting with you. We decided to take a tour with four others to learn the ins and outs of the club. The Cupids were fun and friendly and knew how to rock it. During the tour, I was feeling a tad on edge sexually, from not having seen my man for a while; getting to see the rooms and the dance floor and visualize every incredibly creative thing on my dirty little mind, *Ooh, what I would do …* (Snap! Back to the tour …) Our tour guide gave us glow sticks and told us the only way to get upstairs is with a girl by your side. Even if you came with one, if you go downstairs and decide to come back up, you would be denied! You must have a girl to get in upstairs. And yes, there was a guy at the top of the stairs enforcing this rule. I thought, *Perfect,* as I seductively looked at my date. He responded by pinching my ass, and we proceeded upstairs to five different beds waiting to be played on, each with drapes you could pull across for privacy or leave open for show-and-tell. The beds were deep red in color and leather for easy clean up, plus solid play**. There were baskets of condoms/ supplies at every bed and corner for cleaning up or dirtying up.

In the far-left corner, there was a secluded room with a door and a round bed with intimate lighting. My excitement was driving me wild with lust and sensation and curiosity for other little places as I looked around. We were told that the tower of towels across from this room was for everyone; a card reading "No entry" or "Come watch" was dangling on the doorknob. My date and I smiled while looking intensely into each other's eyes. As we shuffled out into the hall that led to the beds lined up on the left side, adjacent to the stairs, we were introduced to the massage therapist and the rules regarding them. I started looking around the room seductively, imagining every place we could go and what we could do. The tour guide finished showing us that floor and its space, comprised of lined couches against the wall, which was open to all.

We then proceeded to the top floor, passing a hidden bed tucked away in the dark space behind the stairs, as we were led onwards. Seven of us crept up the stairs to the lookout place that went all the way around in a 'U' shape accenting the dance floor. To the right, there was another bed. *Go figure,* I said in my head … and beside that was a closed room that intrigued me. The tour guide opened it up to the dungeon where there was a spank table and a St. Andrew's cross**; my eyes widened to this new profound knowledge. My ideas started getting crazy, and I knew that the upstairs was where we were going to be for most of the night. I squeezed my date's hand and smiled excitedly, but before I could say anything, he said, "The left room is ours." I perked up, not yet knowing what was in that left room. Inside the dungeon was a mini staircase, at the end of which lay a bed prepped for pornographic scenes to commence, lit with the seductive red presence of what was to come. Again, the room could be shut with a mini note stating your preference.

We moved on towards the hall once again and towards my date's favorite room that was saved for last. Our Cupid guide opened the door to a small, room-like closet with a stool and a sex swing.

I giggled, covered my mouth, and smiled at him, immediately longing to start. Everyone shuffled out and thanked the Cupid guide, who was brilliant, might I add. My date and I had gotten the VIP wristband, which included three drinks each and our own "table" (there was no table); the drinks alone paid for themselves, so we didn't mind.

We commenced to the dance floor, pit-stopping along the way to, one: look at one another intensely, and two: draw all over each other with glow paint, or rather I just needed another excuse to touch him while admiring his fit body. I couldn't help but grab a brush and lather neon yellow warrior paint on him; as if he needed more, I drew a heart on his chest and told him how big it was even if he might not know it yet. Then I drew my way down and around, making designs along his muscled arms and thunderous thighs. He quickly grabbed a brush and started painting my ass, tickling me with the cool, thick texture, gliding it up around my waist and along my neck and to my face for warrior-paint markings as well. I threw my lips on his, trying hard to keep our distance till the paint dried.

Putting the brushes down and turning the corner to a stripper pole, *ding-ding!* I suddenly went into dirty slut mode. I whipped off my heels and put a show on for the guys that were sitting around the dance floor, who suddenly tilted in my direction. The pole slid up and down through my fingers, as I gripped hard while spinning around the pole, groping it and torturing the crowd with my sexual energy. I caressed the pole up and down, moving slowly with fiery eyes. I turned around so my plump ass crack could have a slide on the pole, popping it to wiggle for show. Sliding down, I placed my hands over my head, longing for the night to start, and this made me kickstart. I jumped off, wearing a mesmerizing expression, the energy of touch pouring over my body, making my heart beat faster. I looked into my lover's eyes and quickly realized we were dancing and caressing each other slowly to the song as "Faded" came on set. I started kissing his chest and neck, breathing heavy into his ear and on his neck. I creeped my way up, gliding my lips to his so my desires could be met. His soft beard tickled my cheek, and I guided my lips closer to his; as the moment came nearer, he moved my way and met my internal needs. His lips were playful, yet aggressive as we stroked our tongues in each other's mouths, tasting each other's wonders, wanting more. Our bodies were pressed up against each other's beating hearts, racing more and more as we tickled our sensations with our fingertips. Swaying with the beat of the music, it filled our motions, accurately portraying the energy of our feelings towards each other. The background scene started to fade away even though more people made their way over, unaware of the passion and delight they were about to witness.

We looked into each other's eyes like we were lustful, wandering energy fuses that wanted to spark. I swayed with him to the music as the lights danced around us. The floor was ours and I used my hands to feel his dress shirt, untucking it slowly. Between dancing and being engulfed by the night's potion, I reached down to his buttons. One by one, I started to unbutton them. I moved my body up and down his, spinning around him and caressing him as if he were my pole. I kept one hand on him, gliding scantily, the other doing a dance routine with the rest of my body, in motion, moves swaying according to the beats coming over me through the floor. I was putting on a show for on-lookers or maybe it was just for me to enjoy the music moving inside of me.

In my heels, I cat-walked around him, one foot crossing the other. Once I got to his back, I was able to fully take his shirt off. And this shirt did not give any justice to what he had going on underneath. He was impressed and longing for closeness, so he swung me around to face him. I gasped in excitement and giddiness for more. He proceeded to dance and sway with me as he touched me from head to toe; facing me, he moved effortlessly to the floor to drop down low—and low he did with a little nudge into my pussy. She was ready for play and was already dripping from the movements and tension. As he climbed up again, all while kissing and touching me all over, I turned around and popped my ass out while keeping my legs straight and my upper body down to pump and grind. He felt my hips while doing so as I reached around and undid his belt. I turned around and kissed him, nibbling on his lower lip to distract him from the one fell swoop that was his belt coming off. His pants, at that point, weren't a challenge and through the motion of dancing and moving, his pants came off ... And there was me, still wearing all my clothes ... I realized how this must have looked to an outsider. Smiling with accomplishment, I placed his clothes off to the side. When an on-looker questioned, "How did you become undressed, and she didn't?" I smiled and my date replied, "She's that good." At that point, I couldn't hold my desire back and wanted him as much as he wanted me.

The room darkened and our souls were the only ones left with the beat of the music. We stared at each other, snickering amongst ourselves, knowing where to go next. We grabbed each other's hands, forcing our bodies towards what lured us, still capturing each other's wanting eyes. Smiling, I turned around, still holding his hands, and guided him towards the stairs to fully enjoy the night right. While strutting across the floor towards the stairs, everybody glanced over to see the adventurous types go wandering off into sexual bliss. As we were walking up the stairs, I soon realized and wondered if I was dreaming; my eyes shifted to the occupied beds and took in scenes of what you would only imagine in your head. Walking towards bed after bed, I peeped, like a Peeping Tom, to see what act was being displayed. The first bed was closed off; the second bed had one girl and three guys, all naked. The girl was sucking off a guy while lying down, and the second guy was fucking her while semi-standing with one knee on the bed. The third guy was lying next to her, playing with her rear. All I could manage to say was, "Wow," with a slight jaw drop, and behind me, my partner whispered in my ear, "Right!" As his heaving body moved to the last bed to find a threesome of two girls and one guy, his eyes wandered and shifted; he turned his whole body towards me and quickly groped for my hand to lead me towards the bedroom on the opposite side of the space. *Success,* I thought as the place was empty.

We cleaned and prepped our scene**, turning the "Do not enter" sign to "Enter" as I glanced towards him in acknowledged acceptance. I attacked him; waiting for this moment made me realize how much I had been wanting him to take me and touch me all over. We lovingly took our underwear off each other. Mine was done one bra strap at a time, while he kissed each shoulder and pulled the strap between his fingers. His touch made me quiver and moan, and his hot breath seemed to penetrate my skin. He guided his hands down my back to my lovely hips and quickly, without a flinch, threw me onto the round, red leather bed. Wanting him to join me, I wouldn't let go, and I glided my feet against the side of his body towards his sexy "Captain America" underwear. (Sexy, right? He was wearing socks that matched his underwear. Man, I loved his style.) Me, I was in pure white lingerie with white heels and stockings to match. (Why hello, glow party!) His underwear glided right off of his chiseled, muscular body and exposed his excited endowment, showing off how horny he truly was.

He worked his way down my body, badly wanting my naked form against his. I could feel his juicy pre-cum starting to come out of the tip of his beautiful, erect cock as he stroked my body. He kissed my stomach and inner thigh until I was squirming with lust. He slowly moved his hand down in between my legs to caress and test just *how* sexually frustrated I'd become, sweeping my wet pussy with his gentle touch and massaging his fingers inside of me, smiling. His eyes were in a trance. I wriggled and sighed, sneaking my hands towards his inner thigh and, of course, grabbing his ass along the way (and *what an ass*). He thrusted towards me, and I whipped off my panties. He guided his cock towards my slick clit, his tip opening fitting perfectly with my clit. While getting a clitoral massage, I moaned, becoming wetter and wetter by the second. He couldn't resist thrusting a little when he felt the opening; he moaned like no other, wanting more but acknowledging that the time was mine to take. Still, I played with his throbbing cock on my wet, slippery clit, like an instrument wanting the session to start. I teased him, pushing his dick into me more and more, each time playing in between until we both couldn't take the tension. Slowly, I took in every inch as he put his blood-riddled dick into my already sopping wet vagina until we both moaned with power. His dick bottomed out and I gasped. Our heavy breathing filled the room, and we inspired the couples coming to see the show with pleasure. I pulsated with him inside of me, and he showed it on his face, biting his lip and asking how I did that. We sat like that, with him inside of me, so we could feel each other and take a moment to pace and brace for what was to come.

I especially liked it when he threw me around and took charge. He asked me if I was ready; I smirked at him, as if he had to ask. He started slowly and progressed, while I started squirming. My toes curled and back arched the more he moved inside me. When we were in full swing, he buried his face into me and pounded me hard, while I had full view of the door and the excited people watching.

He pulled out and finished on me, filling my belly button with his man protein before he got off to get a towel. Lying there, I knew to clean up. I was exhausted, but I still had room to keep going, so I cleaned and dressed up, and we proceeded back down to the dance floor to mingle and party until we couldn't handle our lust once more and climbed the stairs again to test out the sex swing.

To our amazement, it was free. He quickly plopped me on it, and I laughed when I almost fell out of it backwards. As I braced myself with the straps on either side, he pulled me in and started kissing me, moving down to slide off my white lace underwear once again. He lusciously glided his tongue along my throbbing, ripe pussy. Getting me wet wasn't that hard, but pleasing me was—to the point of climax. I enjoyed every lick and tickle of his beard; pushing myself into him was easy in the swing but made repositioning harder. He came up, wanting me—all of me. I wanted him inside. He dropped his underwear and penetrated me without hesitation this time. Using the swing to his advantage, I could only hold on for the ride. I could feel his throbs of enjoyment as he pulled every inch in and out; I would twitch whenever I felt his dick momentarily on my hard clit. My lips were full and pulsating, but I knew this swing wouldn't do because I enjoyed moving myself; I didn't want to just lie there, taking it.

He loved the swing but could tell I had had enough, and there were other people the swing could serve. Half-naked, we gathered our things and proceeded to the next room—my favorite room— tinted red, closed off, and freedom to move in all positions. After we prepped, he sat up against the headboard and I followed him. Knowing what he wanted, I licked my lips, my gaze piercing his. I asked him if he wanted to know my thoughts, teasing his dick as it grew harder and throbbed at my will. I licked, kissed, and soothed my lips against his shaft, and licked and sucked his balls when I went lower. Feeling his body and hearing his breath as he moaned for more, I grabbed his tight ball sack and played with just the tip of his penis—licking, slowing sucking around, only to prolong his tension. I knew his intention, and pushing me forward was a sign for more. I placed his cock in my mouth, starting with my tongue, engulfing it slowly, ensuring I didn't choke. Then he grabbed my head; I gagged, and my eyes started to water, but I didn't want to stop so I only backed off a bit. I started twist-sucking his dick with my hand, tongue, and mouth, and I grabbed his abs with my other hand to prop myself up. After a few moments, he needed me to stop so he wouldn't blow; he wanted to please me too.

He went down on me once more, at the bottom of the bed, and then pushed me up and threw my leg against the wall for a backwards ass-and-pussy lick. I couldn't help myself—I grabbed his hair and the back of the bed for support. Breathing heavy and tensing up, I let it all out … moaned … panted … released tensed breath and relaxed while my juices ran down his chin and he slurped them up. He told me I tasted good; I smiled and drew him on top of me. He kissed me and threw me around, wanting to just pound me from the back and cum on my ass too. As he pressed forward, he fell into me, releasing.

Wandering back down, exhausted and downing water, the lights were starting to come on. We got invited to an afterparty on the quay, so we went. I asked him, "Was there anyone in the club you were interested in?" He looked at me and said, "Why would I want a piece of the pie when I have the whole thing right here?" He smiled as I melted at his cheesy but sweet statement.

Scott laughed at us on the way to "the Mexican's" afterparty—and yes, they told us to call them that as they were travelling in from Mexico for the party. We chilled and got compliments on our looks, or should I say my BF was getting hit on by the Mexican girl in the room. She asked to make out with him, and right after I said to my BF, "It's your body," he passionately kissed her, and she grabbed his ass. I felt uncomfortable, and the Mexican guy started making out with me. I stopped as I was not feeling it, nor did I feel good doing it. My date was still going at it with the Mexican. After awkwardly waiting for them to finish kissing, I turned around and headed for the door; it was late and the after-afterparty at my BF's place was calling me.

Getting back to his place, I wondered if he was into that Mexican girl, whether he did that with other girls or was just good at getting his way. I pushed my thoughts aside as we stepped inside, walking in to two drunk girls and his roommate. As the music was in full swing, we all started dancing and laughed at the situation. Then we heard noises and ran towards them; Scott and one of the drunk girls were banging, and the girl was screaming with pleasure. He was going down on her, and I could hear them say, "You like that ..." and, "You're sooo yummy," and then, "Get on that couch." I couldn't help but laugh and throw a condom under the locked door after stating, "No fair, I wanted to watch," and jiggling the doorknob.

I went back to dance and helped a drunk girl in the bathroom with her hair. The party soon dissipated, and me and the boy now had the room to ourselves. He led me in. Exhausted, malnourished, dehydrated, and still high, he went on top of me one last time and pounded the last bit of energy we both had out. He pulled out and, to my surprise, hit my face; I laughed and said how impressive that was. I held still; his juices were all over me, covering my body … the slightest movement would soil the sheets.

After cleaning my hair, face, arms, midsection, neck, and legs with a towel, I rushed to the bathroom to wash my pussy and face once more. Lingering in the bathroom, I saw the sun shining. We both passed out, smiling, only to have the smell of bacon wake us up a few hours later. We glanced at each other in remembrance of the night.

# The Learning Curve …

Come open-minded and don't expect anything, PERIOD. This will ease your understanding, mind and body in that atmosphere. I have heard so many people say, "Well, you have to do something there, right?!" NO! In fact, can I get a *HELL NO*?! This is a place for body-positivity, consent culture, community, and so much more. Open your mind and embrace the energy; the first time you go can be just to view, just watch, to maybe only dance on the dance floor downstairs. You do you!

There are a few sayings up in Garden of Eve, including: "Don't be a Creepy Carl" and "Don't be a Touchy Tina." The consent culture there is high standard, more so than at regular clubs, I believe, where I remember getting pulled away from my group by a bunch of guys who grabbed my arm and wouldn't let me go until my friends were in their faces. Here, at Garden of Eve, I have never experienced this, nor have I experienced any unwanted touch at all. If, by chance, this happens, there is an actual process for handling this, which may lead to the guilty party being suspended from the club or blocked. Consent is sexy! Remember that!

A great way to start understanding your yeses and noes is by asking yourself ahead of time. Be mindful and communicate with who you're with or with your partner. The worst is when we go in with assumptions and goals that aren't verbalized, acknowledged, or even checked out to see if they are true/ok. Yikes! It's important to know what touch you're ok with, what play you're ok with—if any—and with whom. It is great to have a foundation in place before any drinking is involved or sexual high you feel towards the party.

The reason behind hiding, nuzzling into your date's neck and not facing each other or looking into each other's eyes could be … well, to focus on them, to hide, to imagine, to … well, a lot of things. Everyone is different on that front. That behavior could be a way of hiding, to not be fully seen by your partner. There are other ways as well, such as turning off the lights to also hide—perhaps to provide cover for your body as you may feel self-conscious about the way you look, move, giggle, or cum! You do you. Be mindful of your whys as this may help you grow.

Boundaries**! Ta-da! The lovely word that is apparently daunting to some, even though we navigate them subconsciously alllll theeee timmmmeee! Asking for someone to do something, rather than asking someone else—boom, boundary! Talking about likes and dislikes, what's ok and not ok … It doesn't have to be big or daunting. Society only puts that out there. There are different forms of boundaries—your *Hell noes!*, your *Maybe we can trys*, and your *Hell yeses!* In common terms: rigid, flexible, and porous. When it comes to this story, we really didn't talk first about the whole kissing others thing. Nor did I think it would have bothered me. I may have been more inclined to shut down the request. The kiss my BF shared with the other woman had me feeling unwanted since he seemed so into it, and I should have verbally said so—I could have said, "I am not ok with this." Either way, I felt icky after. Yes, sometimes you experience "scene blues*."

"Scene blues" happen when you suffer low moments of "Maybe I shouldn't have" style of regret, which again can happen and more often than you would think. There is also sexual compliance*, which happens when you consent to a sexual act you don't really want. Arousal non-concordance* is another state that can complicate being together—this occurs when you experience mismatched physical and subjective (or mental) arousal.

If you don't like something, switch it up. You don't have to like something just because your date does. There might be something "your other" may want to try, and yes, trying is fun! However, if there is a "Heck no, I really don't want to try this," then say so. You have your own personal, unique wants and desires too. Having the exact same set as someone else is unheard of. You will have similarities, but not to the exact tee!

Lastly: Communicate, communicate, communicate. I can't verbalize this enough.

## Glossary

*Arousal Non-Concordance*: Mismatched subjective (or mental) and physical arousal. Basically, your body and your mind are not on the same page sexually in that moment.

*Scene Blues*: Low moments that might feel like regret or an energy dip after a scene happens.

*Sexual Compliance*: There might be times when you say yes to a sexual partner even if you don't particularly feel like having sex. The reasons you might comply sexually when you don't necessarily want to are complex and varied.

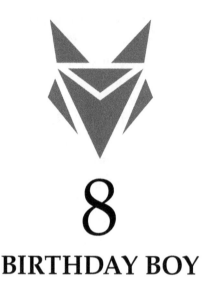

# 8

# BIRTHDAY BOY

~He was the bartender, young and full of charm and charisma. I couldn't stop looking at him and wanting his energy. I wanted all of him and wanted him inside of me.~

*I* was in dire need of something—anything as it'd been close to four months since I'd had sex. The chronic fatigue and pain from an injury I had incurred was cramping my style, especially my libido. I was always thinking about the pain, how tired I was and how most—or everything—hurt on my body at this point. The accident that changed my life knocked me unconscious, gave me a concussion, and chronic symptoms to go with it. I would need something to ease the pain, to wash it away—a drug or something. Anything. Mik gave me a pill. I downed it in the washroom and away I went, after waiting on the sidelines for it to kick in while I polished off some tequila in order to be able to just move. I was self-conscious at this point because I thought others could see the pain, as if I were wearing it on my face. Every step tingled up my body, my mind inflamed and my spirit trying to find the strength to smile.

Mik knew where my head was at; she also knew what to tell me since she had back pain too, of course, in a different sense. She was holding on to intergenerational trauma; She was silently suffering, and it showed up in her body in so many ways. She wanted to help others. It was genuine, but I always wondered if it was a way to dismiss her own pain, a way to look away from her own hurt as it is easier to help than to be helped. She was kind-hearted, with the straightest hair and a kinky spunk to her every move. She was a total ass gal, and she love-love-loved playing and being played with! That was one of her many kinks. She was native, hot as hell, and knew how to party and party well. If you didn't watch out, you'd be up all night and wondering how it happened—all because of this thin, flirty and loving woman. Her tongue ring suited her well; she had many talents, which she was easygoing about offering up to show you.

As the night went on, I kept flirting with the bartender. Mik mentioned it was his birthday while we were sitting on a bench across from the bar. A smile crossed my face as the bartender glanced at me with his twinkling *dare me* eyes. He was handsome, tall, with almost jet-black hair and amazing charm. His smile was welcoming. I bit my bottom lip while talking to Mik. She knew I was numbing my body's pain and that she had to talk close to my ears in order for me to hear past my earplugs. We looked seductive in the presence of onlookers who had no idea what we were talking about. A song we both enjoyed came on, so Mik danced her heart out on the dance floor lit by laser lights, as I bobbed my knees, my feet planted so as not to move or create too much jolting. From afar, it seemed like I was legit dancing a storm. *Little do they know,* I thought.

James was heading my way. My heart pounding, I was flushed and nervous. I could feel the sweet sweat dripping down my back. It was hot down in this underground basement, and mine and Mik's matching police costumes were sexy as hell! I could break the ice and tell him I had to frisk him, maybe handcuff him, maybe question him for processing. *Fuck, he's coming closer.* My mind went blank, and I just said *hey* as he started dancing close to me, asking if it was ok. I nodded; I didn't even say anything. I would've choked on my own words. *Ugh why, V, why?* My girlfriend told me she'd be back—a sassy little feline bouncing around the dance floor had caught her eye. James started kissing my sweat-doused neck that just so happened to mix well with his juicy lips. I closed my eyes as that was the closest someone has gotten to me besides my girlfriend in a while. He whispered in my ear that I tasted like strawberries. I thought I'd be his strawberry kitten for sure. *Pet me all over and make me purr. I'll scratch your back and you'll want it more for sure.* He was delicious—hard and wanting. Pressing into me, I could feel him. I was amazed and wanting. Who was I kidding... I was longing, craving. I had desired this for so long. Having both an angel and a devil on my shoulders didn't help. The angel was about seeking pleasure and the devil was bringing awareness to my pain.

Slowly moving—doing what I could—I caressed, feeling him. He asked if we could do more. I was excited and it showed. I immediately answered with a yes, breathing heavy as my heart kept pounding, thinking about the possibility that his cock was throbbing. I glanced over to see my girlfriend coming back with an ear-to-ear smile. Knowing she'd probably put on a show in the other room, I could feel every inch of my body vibing to the music, to my pussy, to my euphoria. The pain was finally lessening—*bye bye, devil; why hello, pill.* Everything felt so much better; my mind was filled with a lustful serotonin high.

I excused myself to go to the bathroom by telling James to wait there, I'd be right back. I went to freshen up as we had been there dancing around other people and sweating like thieves. I popped a piece of gum and washed my face and down *there.* I wanted to be prepared; I wanted to feel him in me and on top. Looking at myself in the mirror, I took two deep breaths and made sure my false eyelashes were still intact, looking like seductive cat eyes. Next to me, a drag queen said, "Girl, stop. You look amazing. You don't need to be looking so hard." I smiled at her and told her she had made my entire night. Then I complimented her on her skills in super high platform heels. She flipped her hair and popped her side out with a smirk of approval and knowing.

Tumbling out of the bathroom and bracing myself at the entrance, I looked around. James was dancing with Mik, but not close—a safe distance and looking around trying to find me. I thought about how cute that was. Moving slowly towards him, I embraced the slap of heat that hit me as I crossed over onto the dance floor. He instantly kissed me, and wow, was he a kisser. Mik grabbed my ass, and I put James's hand on my ass too, chuckling away as if she had been the instigator. Dang, he could kiss. He was gentle but took me in. We slashed our wet tongues together until Mik broke the silence with "Awww..." I glared at her, as if to say *shut up*. She got the hint and smiled, dancing away with her little feline who had come around to play again.

James slid his hands closer to my throbbing pussy, gently caressing my soaked panties, outlining my pussy lips to my erect clit. I was moaning and kissing him with wonder and delight. I hoped he would ask what I had in mind. I hoped this would last, this wonderful, cloud-like feeling of painless bliss—a wakeful *ahhh...* I bit his bottom lip ever so gently. He slowly backed up and looked at me with a smirk, moving in with more drive and determination, as if I had challenged him. I giggled and moved in closer as well. I could feel his hard dick bulging from his pants as he pressed against my body while we grinded, seeing how much we could handle having a barrier of clothing between us still. He took my hand off his cock and whispered, asking if I would like to go into the next room. Nodding, I was nervous. The next room had a spank table, a viewing area and individual rooms to play in that were very cramped but private. Yes, this was a sex-positive club. I liked putting on a show, but it had been so long. I was nervous, out of practice, and above all, I was with a gorgeous guy I had just met. Talk about a triple threat.

The space was tiny. The club itself was in a basement, with a dance floor, bar/lounge area, viewing area/play and dungeon area. The dungeon area contained a bed and benches; there were condoms, complementary lube, and of course, sanitizing wipes as well. The room we wanted was the one with the spank table in the middle, right next to the bar, separated by a black curtain. The room was dark, but there was enough light spilling in from the dance floor to see by. James took my hand, and as he led me there, I took deep breaths to calm myself, then *bam!* we claimed the spank table. It was free, and there were only two people on the other side of the room. *Fairly empty,* I thought. *Thank God!* I could be an exhibitionist without the pressure.

We started hot and heavy. I barely had anything on, and he didn't want to take his pants off all the way—just to his ankles. I got it—it's hard to get those on and off, especially when you're actually on shift and working, lol... He took my bra off one strap at a time, caressing my boobs; it felt amazing! Everything felt amazing... I felt like I could cum just from a touch. He placed me on the spank table, and I complied. I remained seated while he towered over me, kissing me everywhere, putting his hands all over my sweaty body, gliding with ease. I allowed it all. I was in awe. Moans escaped me as his fingers reached my black lace panties; this time, he moved them aside, accessing my wet, plump lips, ready for him. His fingers glided around in my wetness, first in circles, then in an up-and-down motion, sliding over my erect clit, pushing past my plump lips, making me clench him, wanting him to move in.

My hands on his back, kissing him still, I snapped his belt off with a whipping action. He stopped, and I looked up at him; he had one eyebrow up, as if he was impressed. I smiled as if it was natural and no big deal. I pulled his underwear down with his pants, but he quickly grabbed them, as if I was going too fast for him. I looked at him, questioning. He bent down and said he was shy, that he'd never done anything like this before. I told him I had never done a bartender before, so we were even. I said we could always stop if he didn't want to; he quickly responded with a no and said this WAS what he really wanted, assuming I did too. We proceeded; I put my hands on his cock and glided up and down to get him into it once more—before my abrupt aggressiveness. We continued making out and he went on top of me, feeling me and finally penetrating me with his fingers. He asked how many… I said to start with two and he obeyed. I moaned with pleasure as I hadn't had anyone, not even hands, up there in a while. I had forgotten how it felt, how it pleased me and more.

I could feel my devil coming back; the pill couldn't hold my pain off any longer. He saw it on my face. I told him it was just back pain, and he actually held me up. Others saw and offered a hand; I said sure—only a hand though. An older gentleman helped hold me up while the devil pressed on. I could tell the gentleman got his kicks from watching, and well, that was a great fit then. He was kind. James was still penetrating me with his fingers as I gripped both of them, and wow, was he working me hard. His cock was getting harder just seeing my enjoyment. The sensations were intense, but so was my pain. I tried to just ignore that little devil as long as I could. James asked me for a condom, and I laughed and pointed to the free ones on the wall. He smiled and rolled his eyes to the ceiling, as if saying *oh yeah, duh.* The gentleman grabbed me and held me while James ran over and ran back.

I grabbed his cock and he wrapped it. He asked if I was ready. I leaned back as, at that point, all I could do was slight movement and mostly starfish. My hands were doing most of the work, finding him, gliding his cock towards my slit. He slid it against my dripping wet lips that had been stimulated by his fingers. With a gasp, I felt him finally. I was craving, so I grabbed his ass to move him in even more. He throbbed inside me. We were breathing heavy; he was standing over me, penetrating me, my legs around him. It was slow at first, but then he quicky started to pound me as I asked for harder penetration. I needed the hard, raw, deep kind of sex. The sex you long for and watch porn for—where they just take you and pound you into pleasure. He listened and started going deeper, harder. I pulled back a tiny bit. He asked if I was ok. I nodded, but my back was throbbing, my neck stinging, and my mind was starting to inflate. I ignored my body and just pushed towards my needs and his.

In the middle of it all, I heard someone say, "Thatta boy... Happy birthday!" He continued—smiling, sweating, pounding. I could feel his cock was going to burst, and he didn't last too much longer. I was soaked, head to toe, and so was he. Bent over, he stopped. We both were exasperated and excited to have had that experience. Making out, we put our foreheads together and both said thank you. I slowly got up. He disposed of his condom, wiped off and pulled his white underwear and his sexy jeans up over his well-used dick. He helped me up off the bench and asked if I was ok after thanking the gentleman behind me who had been helping hold me up.

The gentleman said, "No—thank YOU!" with a smile on his face, and James and I went about finding his belt and tee, as he handed my black lace underwear back to me. I was still wearing my black mini skirt and most of my cop outfit. As I came back to the present moment, I looked around and soon realized we had a crowd. They were thanking me and James after they were finished watching us. I flushed with excitement and told James in a whisper, "See? You have groupies!" He blushed and kissed me on the cheek. He asked me again about my back, and I then explained a little more. He was in shock and said he could have been easier on me, so I told him, "That's why I didn't want to tell you." He laughed and I smiled, then he quickly realized he had to go back to the bar. He apologized about the abrupt getaway, and I said, "No worries. We will see each other again." I gave him my number and he went back to work at the bar.

I gathered my mind, slowly walked over to the bathroom to freshen up and see if there were any more devil killers since the devil was killing my angel, my dear desire for pleasure as the pain took over. It was fun, but was it worth the pain? As well as the pain to come days later...

## The Lessons

This is something that is not talked about enough. I didn't even know where to go or who to go to for support/help. I felt alone and no one knew. Others thought I was just out of shape, lazy or simply not interested. I didn't know how to communicate my pain, and I was ashamed of it—ashamed I had to go through this issue, not knowing what to do in a world where, at the time, there were no resources given to me because I hadn't cut open my head; I'd "only" gotten knocked unconscious and was labeled as such clinically. No one was there, and I didn't understand what to do, what to say or how to act. It wasn't till later on that I tried to go out, with earplugs and sunglasses, and after a pep talk.

Sex with the pain was another issue. When your mind is fixed on pain, how can you enjoy pleasure? I used to do a trick where I would pinch myself, somewhere other than where the needle would go, to get my brain to think of that pain rather than the needle pain, if I was getting an IV or blood work. Well, if you're hurting all over, it is hard for the brain to let in pleasure. This happens with stress as well. Your mind is in safety survival mode—why would you procreate when you're in pain? If you're not safe, you shouldn't be trying for any pleasure. That's where the mind goes. Too bad I don't get my kicks from pain. I am not a masochist; it just isn't me. Kudos to those who can. That's how I felt when I was experiencing that level of pain.

In order not to be in agonizing pain all the time, I had to manage pain with substances in an unhealthy way for a while. After having sex with this lovely birthday boy bartender, I was in pain and in bed for days afterwards. My body shut down and said *FUCK YOU!* to me. I had overdone it and it sucked.

However, it's not *not* doable. Being open and honest with your partner can help so that they can navigate and meet you where you're at. You can have intimacy living with pain; it just may take a bit more lead up/help. Talk about pain points, what time of day you may be in more pain, where you experience the most pain, and how to help the other out. Find the best positions. Remember: sex releases endorphins, which decrease pain. Heat, such as that in a warm bath before sex, may help decrease stiffness/pain, as well as stretching. Even exploring different forms of sex may help. Pillows, toys, lube, *oh my!* Explore a little and see what helps you individually.

That said, I kind of didn't have "the talk" with the bartender… oops! We are friends of friends and I have seen him around; however, this is something that was missed. Thank God that in the community we (or should I say I) get tested regularly, so I knew I was clean, and he knew I hadn't been with anyone for a while. Either way, I did have "the talk" after the fact because we did have some more fun with each other till he moved away. Bye, James!

For the people who have to deal with pain in your everyday lives and in your sexy lives, I feel ya. SERIOUSLY. This isn't talked about enough because we are supposed to have sexy, spunky, lively sex like we see on TV. (Just joking!) However, more and more people with chronic issues do have to deal with pain and understanding the coping strategies around it. For those that do, I applaud you.

Stay safe, stay sane, stay seen.

## Glossary

*Sex-positivity*: Normalizing sexuality for pleasure as a consent culture.

*Exhibitionist*: One who likes to put on a show; essentially, finding pleasure from being watched.

*Masochism*: The practice of deriving sexual pleasure from pain; a masochist is one who gets turned on by being hurt.

*Starfish*: A sexual position where one essentially lies like a starfish, wide open in the missionary position as a bottom, hands and legs spread so the other person has to do all the work.

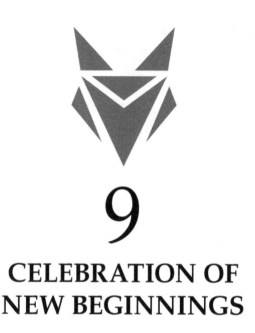

# 9

# CELEBRATION OF NEW BEGINNINGS

-He asked me to introduce him to the lifestyle. I said, "Give me your weekend and I'll do the rest," and he replied, "Done!" Knowing what I was going to do for him and where, I had a wide grin on my face. He responded, "Umm … What did I just get myself into?" Smiling with a slight laugh, I said, "No backing out now." He had no idea the ride he was about to get on.-

He had never gotten into the scene I was into, so he was cautious but curious at the same time. Knowing I was into these types of scenes helped his nerves. Letting me take him by the hand was my personal specialty. I loved introducing people to the community and loved that my friend Vlad had come to me for just that. He entrusted me with his weekend and this weekend was not just for fun, play**, and new adventures; it was the first weekend he and his girlfriend had officially moved on and out of each other's lives. Now on to the fun …

I knew I wanted to start his weekend with a big bang, and so I did. I scheduled two play parties and even made his costume for the first. I made sure he was covered for both events; the first, he volunteered as a Cupid with me so he could meet and greet people and quickly make friends in the scene as well. The second party, well … I'll save that one till we get there …

The first night, Vlad was a newcomer, and we were off to The Dungeon downtown. He lived close by, so I came over to dress him and prep him for the event. It was Alice-in-Wonderland themed, and I was the *Cheshire* Cat—the naughty fishnet version—and he was the White Rabbit. I made him fur cuffs and bracelets, a pair of ears and a tail, and topped the whole ensemble off with a pocket watch that went nicely with his black vest and black underwear. It was early and still bright out, but we didn't care. Walking down Rainbow Street while the little kids said, "Look, Mom, a rabbit and a cat!", no one even thought twice about it as Rainbow Street was anti-discrimination, showcasing all walks of life, which I loved.

He was nervous, but I skipped and giggled, excited for what the night would bring. We arrived early so I could give him a tour of the place and introduce him to everyone there. I explained that the bathrooms were unisex, the dungeon had a monitor**, there were glory holes, beds, sex swings, a Sybian machine*, and spank tables. This club offered a good introductory to the scene as everyone was welcome, we could volunteer to meet everyone, and it was only one floor.

Putting on our wings for our Cupid duties for the night, I described what we would do: Greet, give tours if requested, answer questions, report misbehavior, and make sure everyone picked up a green "go" card or a red "no" card in the process. On the card, you could write your play preference, your kink** (if any), who you're looking for, and your name. It was entertaining viewing the preferences of different individuals and what people wanted from one another. One had a green card with their Dom** name on it; "Xan" was looking for a sub** with a booty to tame.

Vlad picked it all up fast. The more people that came in, the more dressed up the scene became and the more open-minded he became too. The only one I wanted to know was the bartender, since I tended to have good luck in that department. I made friends fast, plus free drinks weren't bad. Our shift was over and now that we knew half the people in there, it was easier for Vlad to relax a bit. Still, the nudity and outfits, men-on-men action, and sex-on-the-premises play was overwhelming, so we decided to take another peek around as the night was bumping. My lovely friends D+M were going at it on the sex bench in plain view. We high-fived him and gave her a kiss as we passed; she was getting pounded doggy style, fitting as she was his pet and on a nice leash, complete with ears. D was a hot little number and M was her master*; they loved each other, and it showed. Vlad just looked at me wide-eyed as I waved for him to come forward into the dungeon. Instantly, he was at a loss for words; everything was being used. The Sybian machine was getting the ride of a lifetime, and the faces its occupants were making made me want to hop on. Our faces beamed as we surveyed the room and Vlad could only let out a slight breath. For him, it was sensory overload. I said, "Welcome to my life," with a big smile on my face, and he looked at me and chuckled, his eyes wide with wonder. He seemed not to know where to look next, or if he should. He needed air ...

Moments later, we reconnected, but first, I left him to wander and explore. While I danced around, I eyed the bartender and leaned in. "When are you off?" I asked. He smiled and said, "Actually, soon." I told him I'd save him a dance and smiled as I turned to the dance floor. It was dark and loud, and the lights fell in with the music. No wonder I loved this place, and it was a good place for someone just getting into it as well. In the back, I knew rope play could be found. In the front, I saw D+M going at it by the dance floor. I also saw Vlad, wide-eyed, jaw to the floor. He was speechless.

I moved towards him and said, "HOT? Right?" He rolled his eyes and sucked in air as if to say he needed to acknowledge how hot it truly was.

Dancing with him, we got close. I could feel his dick getting turned on, but he didn't know how to hide it well, as it was his first time here and he didn't fully know how to act. He said in my ear, "If you're going to dance with me like that, that's gonna happen so … sorry." I laughed and said it was a compliment that he was getting turned on. He looked relieved. I turned around and went down low— dirty and deep, just like the bass. After a while, he found another girl and my bartender got off. We danced and I started making out with him. Vlad said, "That was fast," to the both of us. I said, "Yes, we don't waste time." The bartender whispered in my ear that he had never done this before. I squinted at him and said, "Danced with a girl?" He laughed and said no, he'd never made out with a girl he'd just met. I smiled and said, "Well, there is room for more firsts tonight." Feeling sly and on fire, I kept it up and we played around, touching and fondling. I teased his cock as it got hard. He closed his eyes every so often from the pleasure I was intoxicating him with. He turned me around and bumped and grinded against me while feeling me up. I moved his hands lower.

We had fun, but my friend was there with me, and I couldn't leave him for long. I decided to break free and check in. I slid over to the bar where Vlad was and said, "Hey!" Surprised at how fast I was, he looked over and I smiled and said, "That was nothing." He let out a deep breath and we went for air. Looking around, I knew it was time for us to part with the night; the scene was thinning, and the time was ticking. We had another night coming up. Saying our goodbyes, I got invited back next week by Mr. Bartender. We practically hopped and crawled out, kissing goodbyes to everyone I knew.

Walking home, I could tell something was off. I had kissed Vlad when we were dancing, but he wasn't used to such a forward nature. Back at his apartment, I tilted my head while decorating a tree on my tippy toes with glow-in-the-dark bracelets and asked what he had on his mind. He looked at me and said, "I don't know how to say this but," he took a big breath, "I hope you don't think anything more will happen tonight." I stopped and looked at him, confused, the side of my lip curled up. "What is that supposed to mean? What was happening?" I asked. He looked at me and said, "Well, we got close, and I don't want you to think I was leading you on ..." I smiled and said, "You do realize I was making out with the bartender ..." He looked at me, still wanting clarity. I went over to him. "Don't worry. There is nothing more here. We are friends, and by this weekend, we will be great friends," I said with a gleaming smile. He looked at me, curious, and I said, "One down ... One more to go!"

After a refreshing cat nap (Pun, LOL! Because I was a cat ... no? Fine ... ANYways), I got ready for the next adventure—Garden of Eve. I was to meet Vlad at his place again and dress him, and then we would all go there. Oh, yeah, this time another girl was coming with us ... Let's call her "Trish." Trish was adorable and full of life. At this point in time, loud music while playing dress-up was a must. And off we went in lingerie and neon fishnets, complete with big Asian fans in hand.

Singing Backstreet Boys and old school tunes, we booked it to adventure number two. On the way, I gave them the lowdown ... well, more for Vlad as Trish was in the scene already. I explained about the rules, the rooms, and the floors. He looked at me as if he was trying to wrap his head around what to expect. I told him not to expect anything. When we got there, he watched the video, signed the wavier, and went off for the tour. After that was done, his mind was on overload; the night was already in full swing on the dance floor and soon to be upstairs as well.

The place had three floors and eye candy all around. He whispered, "Thank you," in my ear, but I told him to hold that till the end because the night had just begun. Smiling, I went for drinks and proceeded to the dance floor as onlookers viewed the two new babes that had come in. Vlad was in awe. With two beauties by his side, he was gleaming.

He said that going to the first club was a great intro since this place was bigger and had a lot more play space. Some of the main differences were: bottoms had to be covered on the dance floor, sex/play was only allowed upstairs, drinks weren't permitted upstairs either, and you needed a woman to get you up there.

Saying hi to people I knew and introducing Vlad and Trish, I was dancing hard and getting asked to play. Then Trish saw the pole and off she went. I didn't know what she would do, but she owned it. I sat down and she gave me a private show with her eyes before stopping to give me a not-so-private lap dance for all to see. I had to use our big fans as it was hot, and she was heating me up as well. Vlad was in amazement and couldn't stop staring as she flipped upside-down and twirled around with ease. I was in awe. He closed his eyes and put his hands in front of him, trying not to get hard. After Trish was done on the pole (Note to pedestrians: Do not cross where legs are flying around a pole … you will get hit by a heel … oops!), I asked them both if they wanted to wander. Vlad wanted me to take the lead, so I did. I knew from an earlier conversation with Vlad that there was something on his bucket list that I could help him with (even though he didn't know it yet), so I asked Trish if she wanted all three of us to check out upstairs. We went hand-in-hand upstairs and looked around the first floor. It was packed. Once again, Vlad was in amazement and experiencing sensory overload. There were guys with one girl, girls with one guy, couples, swingers* galore, and more. Some curtains were open for viewing and some were closed for privacy. To the right, guys were going down on girls and guys were getting head; everywhere you saw nakedness and heard the sounds of pleasure. Vlad was in disbelief, so I grabbed his hand and we proceeded upstairs.

Upstairs, the orgy bed was bumping. When I turned towards my favorite room, I smiled because it was open and unused. *Perfect,* I thought. "The universe is giving us a sign," I said. "My favorite room

is free." Vlad asked, "Why is this your favorite?" First off, the red
light, but also the loud music, and the ceiling and walls were close
for anchoring oneself in fun positions. It was also warm in there,
comfortably so. I smiled with a toothy grin. We went inside.

Since I was gonna be the lead, I started kissing Trish and
undressing her. I moved Vlad closer and kissed him. (Yes, we had
cleaned the bed beforehand.) He was shaking so I stopped and
looked at him, asking, "Why are you shaking?" He said he was
nervous. I told him to close his eyes and think of the music, think
of the amazing, blissful beats. "It's only you and me. No one else."
He breathed deep, in and out through his month. He did it three
more times before opening his eyes and fixing them on me. I said,
"Stop over thinking it. Don't expect anything. Just let things happen
as they will." He nodded and started to relax his tense muscles and
overactive mind. "Just BE," I said. "Be here, in this moment, in the
present and enjoy it." Smiling, he nodded again and said, "Thank
you," with a big breath. And so the night began ...

The music bumped and buzzed about the room, the heat causing
our clothes to slide off. It was the three of us and what a gorgeous
time it was. Trish was amazing; her clit lips were tiny and tight. I
began licking her, playing and nuzzling my face in her pussy as she
let out animal growls. Lying beside her, Vlad let out growls to match
as he kissed and caressed her. I stopped and teased that we were in
a jungle, chuckling as they both growled at each other.

We slowly undressed him and slipped off our lingerie, unaware
of who was unbuckling what at this point, since everyone's hands
were everywhere, helping one another out. Trish and Vlad were
following my instructions; it was hot. I motioned where each should
go and place what where. Then I told Vlad it was his turn as I got
up from in between Trish's legs. Moving up to her round, natural
breasts, I kissed her inner thighs. I licked and nibbled, switching
between each breast. Her eyes were closed, her expression consumed
with lust. She was enjoying herself, letting her wild beast come out to
play. I was enjoying her movements while Vlad was making her purr.

He was growling on her pussy, causing a vibrating buzz on her clit. She squirmed from all this pleasure; he placed his hands on either side of her outer thighs and moved her closer to his face, spreading her apart for ease of access. I wanted her to shake so I started playing with her clit and kissing her as Vlad tongued her and grabbed her ass. She was in true ecstasy; her movements became firmer and more insistent. I smiled as she moaned and trembled, both of us blissful from all the action.

I quickly told Vlad to move to the head of the bed and sit on the ledge. He was feeling exposed and wondering what he was doing, so I started licking and kissing his cock, average-sized and easy to engorge fully in one's mouth. Trish was kissing him, and then I guided her down to his cock as well. Looking up at him, I could see what he was thinking: "Holy fuck, this is hot!" I smirked, knowing that this fantasy had been on his list—two hot girls going down on him. *Check*! I said in my head. Trish and I were both tonguing his cock and teasing him, and it was hard for him to handle, so he wanted to play with both of us some more. Before long, I didn't have to tell them what to do; they had caught the flow, and we switched it up—Vlad down on me, Trish on him, and me on Trish, making a spiral flower. We swapped once more before the room got too hot. Sweat dripped in our eyes; we needed air and our parched throats needed water. We decided to take a break. When we opened the door, the song "I Just Had Sex" came blaring into the room. We all looked at each other and laughed, and I said, "How fitting."

We descended the stairs, grabbed some water, and looked out over the dance floor. Trish and I got approached by a man who wanted us to fool around with his new fiancée. We looked around and laughed, wondering if she truly existed. Since we didn't see her anywhere, we asked where she was. He asked if we were together, and of course we said yes and followed him to the sex swing where she was. It was cramped so I suggested we move to a bed for more room. So we all went downstairs to the second floor, and low and behold, a room was free. Vlad was behind us, wondering what was going on. I explained and asked the couple if he could watch. They agreed as long as it was just the girls playing and the two guys watching.

As the fondling and playing progressed, we discovered the fiancée had a torturous wrap-around piece on that was like a puzzle you had to figure out before you could get it off. Laughing, I tried to find where the thing ended and began; the laces were all over the place. Trish was helping, but then the BF said screw it, he would buy her another, and ripped it off of her. That put me a little on edge; I said we would eventually get it. She said, "Whatever," like she wanted to move past it and so did I.

As we moved forward, her BF moved in. He asked his fiancée if it was alright if he and Vlad joined in. She looked up and said it was ok, so we all started playing. Two guys, three girls. Since I was the only one with experience in this play session, I was checking in and calling the shots, making sure everything was consensual, and that the fiancée was fine with her BF nearly fisting me and with me loving it. I was howling with pleasure. He was holding me close, telling me to say certain phrases, like "Tell me you like it … Tell me you want it … Tell me *more* … Tell me *harder*." I repeated everything he said and enjoyed every moment—except when I noticed that he'd forgotten to pay attention to his fiancée. I stopped and asked her again if she was ok and she said yes. I told him to pay attention to her. He just asked her if she was fine; of course she said yes, and he pressed forward with me again, pounding my pussy with his hands and holding me down so I could take it. I gasped as I came hard and made sure my noises communicated as much. Squealing, I released. He then moved over to Trish for more play and started going down on her while she was eating out his fiancée.

Vlad noticed and said, "You looked like you were having fun." I smiled and nodded as he nervously kissed the BF's fiancée while fondling her big boobs as they bounced to the rhythm of the oral train at play. Vlad came closer and I sucked him off.

Soon enough, Vlad was standing, wanting water and so did I. The lights were starting to come on, and the cleaners were starting to clean up. As we were parting ways, I noticed one of the cleaners glaring at me. It was him—the dick. Side note: I went on a little outing with him to see if we matched, and he made fun of me, said he could do my job, and acted like a little child the whole time. We were not a match. And at that particular time in my life, I was so stressed out that sex or play was not on the table either and that's what I had told him. After he saw me playing tonight, he spazzed out, saying how I was such a lying piece of shit bitch … blah blah blah … to which I told him to never speak to me again and that I would be blocking him from now on. Needless to say, I knew something was off about him but couldn't put my figure on it. I had just trusted my gut. THANK GOD for my gut.

Shaken up, I made it downstairs. We were parched and hungry, eyeing the table spread for assembling mini sandwiches and the gallons of water. I was in heaven and had a food orgasm—we all did.

Back at Vlad's, we had a mini after-party, with water, foot rubs, chats, shower rubdowns, and naked cuddling. The morning brought Vlad a reason to smile—waking up to two gorgeous naked women on either side of him. I said, "See, now you can check that off your buck list …"

## The (Double) Night's Lessons

*Don't ask for my help unless you trust me enough to be willing to go full on.* Once you give me your weekend, I have it. And I will make it worth your while. Knowing this, I knew he would have a great time and I was already envisioning the second night. The first night, I had to warm him up in order to find out where his boundaries** were. Having the chat about intentions is the best way to know where you stand, even as friends. Understanding where the boundaries lie can minimize the need for guesswork and make everything so much easier and less complicated.

*Ask and you shall receive.* You want to go to a play party? Perfect!

Let's do it. You want me to take the lead? Awesome! I will make it happen. If you show me your bucket list, I will check some of them off (insert: smirk). Yes, I tend to make things happen. It's in my nature, my essence, and I had been learning to channel it more and more. But if you don't ask, or don't tell me your desires, it won't happen because I won't know to even try. Share your wishes, your desires, your wants and needs. Because once you communicate your intentions, amazing things start to happen ... and that amazing thing is me, Zara! *Cough, cough*—just joking!

*Presence is important.* We make up stories in our head about what's going on and listen to different scenarios about what might happen. GET OUT OF YOUR HEAD! Yes, that's right—stop thinking and just BE. By just *being*, we come back to the present. The most common way to come back into the moment is to focus on one's breath or heartbeat. Once you've tuned into your internal oneness again, we can go back to cultivating the present moment. Enjoy it and relax into sweet, sweet ecstasy. The point is to enjoy the moments as they come without worrying about their meaning. Be in the now.

*Regular check-ins!* With the fiancée and the BF, I didn't tell you she was upset later on. When we were all back downstairs afterwards, she was glaring at him while he complimented me. It looked like she was crying, and now he was the jerk who had to console her and make her feel safe, something she badly needed. She wasn't feeling wanted enough and/or she just didn't speak up while we were all playing together. Either way, their communication broke down and that's why check-ins while playing are so important. We did have the conversation, and she went along with everything, but even though she was in the wrong for not communicating her true feelings, he was in the wrong for not checking in with her as well. Be on the safe side: check in and do it frequently.

*Trust your gut.* You know that crazy guy you went on one date with and now he won't leave you alone when you're busy? Yes, him. Well, he was at the club that night. He works there and trash talks.

Trusting my gut and pulling back was a smart move, and I dodged a bullet (*wipes forehead*). I didn't tell you this, but as I was getting my friends into the club, he was trying to get my attention so we could talk, and I told him I wasn't going to have time. He acted like a little child and kept it up by giving me extra glow sticks and butting in when I was chatting with my friends. Even though that was his way of trying to be nice, I am not interested in being a babysitter to an adult, especially one who already dissed me at our first meeting. Listening to your intuition is super important, for women especially. Trust yourself. Because, if not you, then who?

Foot rubs … Yes … That's all I have left to say …

# Glossary

*Master*: A master is the one who calls the shots, with the consent of the submissive person who calls them such. Masters are often dominant and stern.

*Swingers*: Couples who have consensual sexual relations with other couples.

*Sybian machine:* A device you ride on that has different attachments with different speeds. Usually used for female masturbation, it can be for oral play and a fun way for couples to experiment with the speed dial.

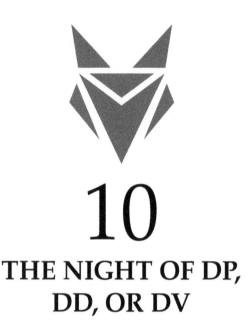

# 10

# THE NIGHT OF DP, DD, OR DV

~He was longing for me to have two guys at once, and I wanted to submit to his desire. I never tried a DD but had experienced DP—just not this kind. This kind you don't know what to call, but it makes a great story and an even better "Best Friends Forever" type of play. THIS was the afterparty … ~

The night was no other than Garden of Eve's famous event. It went off without a hitch. Hot and steamy, the night took us away. The lights came on slowly as we wandered and gathered, thirsty for more.

Constellation was across the street. It was old school, vintage, and full of club-goers. Still dressed to impress, we stumbled across the way and shushed each other through the back door. We creeped up the creaky old wooden stairs to the third-floor rooms for more play**. Other people from the club had rented rooms on the same floor for some more fun after the club. When we wandered in, we knew the vibe was right up our alley. Fifteen of us were in full swing, play bags open, gear out, snacks and drinks on the table near the doorway, and open play spaces for us to figure out how to fill.

To our left, the first bedroom was for play, and the bedroom on the right was for sleeping, lights out, and quiet only. This was a room for couples who had been together for a while—married and in the scene. Xavier and Rebecca were all into dress-up—their usual Mad Max theme. Trust me when I say they dress up to dress down, with layers upon layers to remove as the night progresses—from black eyeliner, black fishnets, and leather to vintage top hats and spiked goggles.

After exploring more, I knew this was gonna be a long night. I hung out and said hi to everyone before whispering to Tristan that I was gonna go freshen up. The bathroom was by the front door, and inside of it was a clawfoot tub to go with the vintage retro décor. After finally realizing that I was supposed to pull down the toilet handle to flush, I looked in the mirror and laughed at how long it had taken me to figure that out. My eyes were batty, my skin flushed. I patted my face with tissue to reduce the shine and reapplied some deodorant, all while giving myself a pep talk ... "Z, you're ok. No expectations. Just go with what feels right, right now." Taking a deep breath, I smiled, thinking that was all I needed.

When I exited, I ran into other people I knew, and soon, the room got busier and busier. More clothes were coming off, and the love language* of touch was lavished on us all. Once I got back to the playroom, my eyes went wide. Sarah (who was Intersex* and wow, was she beautiful) was lying in the middle of the bed with five people around her. Darius was sucking her off; another, while getting licked on the side, was nibbling on Sarah's left breast, and the others were fondling away at each other. Sarah was kind, gentle, and full of wonder, and everyone wanted to embrace her energy. She was beautifully born with both parts, which gave her more things to play with. I wanted her. I was intrigued, and I wanted to play—to suck on her boobs and kiss her while Darius was sucking her off. Sarah was the goddess of this night, lying on her back in the middle of the bed, letting us devour her.

I asked if I could come and watch. Looking into her doe eyes, I sat while she seduced me with them. Tristan was in the other room, chatting. He loved to see me in my element—feeling free and having fun. This is what he wanted every night. Sarah had a cool ease to her. It was seductive. Her look and the way she bit her lip while watching others play and sway made me want her even more. I asked her if we could do some light petting—if I could maybe even touch her boobs. With a smirk, she replied, "I thought you'd never ask!" Excited, I dove in. Getting to touch her silky white skin instantly amplified all the happy pills and drinks swirling in me. It was almost as if I knew her body and skin—refreshing and somehow comforting at the same time, as if we had a past but had never had the chance to indulge.

My hand brushed her skin, towards her boobs, and she loved it. She pressed into me, breathing heavy as I looked deep into her exotic brown eyes. I looked down at Darius, who was servicing her, and he was loving it as much as she was. Her cock was average in length, but her girth was outstanding. Darius gushed a bit from the sides of his mouth while sliding her in and out, popping with suction at the tip. Sarah went in to kiss me, but I pulled away a bit. Because of the dynamic of my own relationship, we did not kiss others. I found it too intimate and wanted that to stay between Tristan and me. I leaned in close and told her. She smiled and brushed up against my parted lips to tease me about what I was missing out on. I closed my eyes, gulped, and bit my lip. When I opened my eyes again, I smiled back.

Suddenly, there were more people in the room, and my bestie was one of them. She was a firecracker with purple hair and waves for days. She was the energy I had been missing since my accident. She was bouncy and full of life! Thankfully, she had enough for us both. She was loaded up with a toy bag full of goodies, and she whipped out a big strap-on dildo to smack me with. It startled me, but only a little because I knew her personality, and it was her style to do just that. I giggled and smiled at her, asking, "What ya thinking you're gonna do with that?" "Oh, YOU know!" she said with a smirk and an evil laugh. She was my Master**, and she knew how to bind me good.

While she unpacked, I looked down the bed and saw Mallory and Ryan going at it on the bottom corner. Mallory looked at the strap-on with curiosity when my Master put it down. Picking up the thickest cock she had, my Master asked Mallory, "You wanna?" Mallory said, "Well …" in a raspy voice that was sexy. "Hold on. I was curious, but let's start slow and ease into it. Maybe not …" My Master cut her off, saying, "Oh, yeah no! This one's for her," and pointed the dildo at me. I smiled.

Mallory bounced up in relief and said, "Ok, lets do this!" Thinking she had more time to warm up, my Master was caught off guard. "Give me a sec," she said. Mallory replied slyly, "I thought you were the queen and master." Master cocked her head, "Oh, you're gonna get it now. Bend over, bitch." Mallory popped her ass up in the air. Master said, "Well, shit, you're tall." She grabbed a chair and said, "This is a first …" At first, it was awkward; Mallory kept servicing Ryan while getting pounded by Master from the back, but she laughed, and soon the train and rhythm were impressive. After a bit, I was beside Mallory, getting pounded by Tristan. Oh, how he could get my body to crave more! His dick was delicious. My sex was vibrating and swollen. Mallory and I getting pounded beside each other must have been quite a sight—after all, we did have an audience now.

Moments later, Brooklyn (my Master) needed a break and tapped me in. It was my first time with Mallory, and she eagerly consented to it all. Brooklyn strapped me in, gave me guidance, and straight up told me what to do. It was awkward for sure. I needed a chair—more like a half-chair, something that hasn't exactly been invented LOL. I had one foot on the chair and the other on the ground while I pounded her from the back and grabbed her hips to press her further into me. It was hard to balance and the rhythm hard to focus on. Even with her butt above the bed, my 5'8" stance still had no chance. I tiptoed, squatted, side-stepped, even fell a bunch of times. Yes, I fell off the chair and laughed my ass off (so did everyone else). I pressed till she and I were out of breath. She couldn't even service her man anymore because the pounding was knocking her forward, hitting the mark. This was our version of a DP*. In a way, it was a "double penetration" because Mallory had gotten a pounding from two girls. Booyah! I think that's one helluva achievement.

Quenching my thirst by getting my Master to do her work on me was my goal. I flirted, teased, and was being a brat* (not really—I just wanted her to "punish" me. To get her to flog**, slap, and pound me). I was wet, willing, and wanting. On all fours, I was begging her to start. She pulled out the big one, strapped it on, and slowly penetrated me. She glided it in at first, and I shivered with passionate delight. I had been itching for this. After I was gushing, she gave it to me hard, and I grabbed the corners of the carpet and moaned harder and harder. All the while a crowed watched. I didn't know—I was in a pure state of bliss.

Tristan slid on to the ground in front of me and said, "Wow, that's hot." He loved watching me get fucked. It didn't matter if it was by a guy or by my Master; seeing me in pleasure was what he loved. The dildo was big like Tristan, and it held its strength, pound after pound. The rush and adrenaline were filling me, pleasing me beyond and then some. I came and continued to have more orgasms, as a circle formed on the sidelines. One woman was in the middle of six men, servicing them one by one in a row, like in a porno. I thought to myself how this was just another night to me, but for others, it would have taken place only in a dream world they would never discover.

Brooklyn did me till I couldn't handle any more. The combination of my noises, my sex, the erotic ecstasy—all had sent my endorphins soaring. I was horny as hell and needed more. Since I was exasperated and thirsty, Tristan gabbed some water for me as I moved over to him for a break. My Master said, "Good girl," and, "That's my girl," while she petted my head, and I nuzzled in, satisfied. The hard wood floors had started to irritate my knees; the carpet only covered so much, and every pleasurable pound had sent me forward. Starry-eyed and experiencing sexual euphoria, I looked back at my Master, depleted. My breath was heavy and panting. My body throbbed, and my abs were sore from the tension. "Break!" I exhaled. After my Master released me, I crawled over to the food and water table. My Sir* (Tristan) petted me with delight. He was craving, wanting his turn to devour me.

On the floor, we passionately kissed, grinding our sweaty bodies together, wanting more. After a while of this lovely wet foreplay and Tristan licking his way towards my inner peace, he slid in front of me and asked if I wanted to try DV* (Double Vagina). Facing him, our bodies still entwined, I hemmed and hawed. But looking at him and looking around the room, I thought this would be a good time; the crowd had thinned, and my pussy was primed. I asked with who, and Tristan pursed his lips and said Greyson was willing and interested. Plus, he had volunteered immediately. Greyson then asked his intimate partner, and they sat on the couch, talking. Tristan had his in, so we briefly chatted, and Tristan (my Sir!) gave *me* a puppy-eyed please of a smirk, complete with a twinkle in his eyes. I had never done this before, so I thought, *Why not?* My Master had already warmed me up, surely this wouldn't be that much more? Boy, was I wrong.

Since it was my first (and maybe my last) time, I didn't know how to proceed, so I asked Tristan to navigate. I would give it a try even just for the sake of it. Greyson was average sized, and were he any bigger, I would have gotten hurt. Tristan was girthy and big in all the right ways, with a slight bend up. He navigated from the bottom while I straddled him from on top. Greyson was behind me. He was handsome and kind-looking, tall and fair with salt and pepper hair and a killer smirk. And he had warm, comfortable energy to top it off, nothing like the mystery Tristan had in that twinkle in his husky blue-grey eyes.

Getting them both in, making room with a slight rhythm, was a slow and steady process. Tristan was super sore since he had been pounding me on the floor earlier. His body reacted to the other guy's essence and my pleasure, and he knew I was his—all his—to play with. His dick was overpowering the other guy's dick. Tristan's intensity and size moved Greyson out of me. My vagina was not loving it—two dicks stretching me beyond my max was overkill. As we tumbled and fumbled slowly, they took the lead. I could barely move in my position, and I was scared I would hurt myself. We laughed, we tried, we re-arranged, but Tristan kept filling me up, leaving almost no room for Greyson. After a little while, we actually got some rhythm down, but I thanked them both for the experience. They were smiling end-to-end, saying, "Yes!! Thank you!!" At least I tried it, and maybe I would again with a smaller guy …

The experience of another guy touching me, pounding me, had Tristan incredibly turned on. He had to take me for himself. We had sex everywhere after that, our third (or maybe fourth) wind fueled by passion and lust. We were putting on yet another show (or more like a *showstopper*) for all to see. As the night became morning, we finally started to burn out. When the sun came up, we decided it was time for our bodies to breathe, rest, and reset. We must have had sex at least 12 times that night.

## The Lessons

Well, that was an experience for sure. Nothing swung the wrong way, nor was there a part of me that thought, *Crap!* The only thing that might have benefited the situation more was if my Master had been there navigating the DV and watching it unfold. I had never done it before, nor do I think I am likely to again. For future reference: If you have a tight vagina, you may want to go with smaller guys or even just do DP.

Remember to stay hydrated. And clean up afterwards, not just yourself, but any tools or equipment you might have used too.

And two words: rest and reset.

As far as relationship dynamics go, everyone has their own. Never, NEVER! assume someone else's just because of the label they carry, such as "monogamous" or "polyamorous"*. In my relationship, we struggled at first because, well, there were differences in what we each thought was ok and not ok. Boundaries** were crossed because of a lack of communication and loving, open-ended questions working towards such things like boundaries. Needless to say, we learned, and he learned *hard*. We have check-ins and ask (if we really want to try something), as well as aftercare** where we talk about what maybe worked or didn't work. For example, the kissing—Tristan thought he could continue kissing others even though we were in a relationship, and he did so without really chatting with me first to see if I was ok with it. Later on, we realized—or shall I say, *he* realized—after a not-so-fun fight that kissing others was a no-go for me. We struggled to adjust for a little while; he acted out like a child, saying I couldn't "tell him what to do." Really, I hadn't been *telling*—I had been trying to *collaborate*. He had needs too that I had consented to.

Relationships should be a dance, not a tug-of-war. This was the first relationship where I had felt all the things—the "long-term" pin in my brain; how I didn't want to lose him; and how kissing was actually something that was very intimate with him (yes, he is an amazing kisser, among other things). He was way more open than I was. In the past, I had always been the open one in my relationships, but with Tristan, I got triggered a lot at first—as one would with a person they deeply care for. When you get triggered like this, you risk losing someone amazing too.

I opened up the conversation about boundaries and shared how I was feeling about all of it. He had a hard time initially since he was no guru when it came to, of all things, communication and boundaries. From there, we experienced slip-ups, few and far between, and self-sabotaging behaviors that also affected our relationship. However, talking through them and validating the other's pain and hurt by acknowledging them and owning up/ taking responsibility really helps. We can't change the past—we are human—but we can invest in our future and learn from our mistakes and take precautions when moving forward and rebuilding.

Some of you may be wondering what's up with this "Sir" and "Master" business? Well, I'll give you a breakdown. My Master is the one that controls the situation when I'm in a scene**. She has total consent, and I can always stop or say no. My Sir is my man, my guy, the one and only, the primary in my life. We kinda like playing with the idea, and so far, we love it. My Sir doesn't get called that all the time—only when we are playing. He is gentle, but he has a strong, dominant presence to him. My Master, on the other hand, has more of a role in punishing me when I get out of line or if I tease her in our scenes. I submit to my Master when we are in scene, and she is stern with me. They both play their roles well, and I get to play the submissive** with each of them, which is something that I enjoy and something that also turns me on.

Lastly, one more word: Ask!!! Always ask questions and do not hesitate to take a break. You are there for you.

# Glossary

*Brat*: In the lifestyle/kink community, "brat" is a term used when someone wants to be put in their place by a master, Dom, or tamer. Brats act out almost like teenagers and receive "punishments" in return. Most importantly, this is all consensual.

*DP (Double Penetration)*: Usually, this involves one woman consenting to penetration from one guy from the front (vagina) and one penetrating her from the back (butt), a.k.a. "One in the pink and one in the stink," but—that expression sucks, so please don't use it.

*DV (Double Vagina)*: DV happens when a woman takes two cocks in the pussy at the same time. DP is sometimes used in lieu of DV.

*Intersex*: A person born with both reproductive or sexual parts, an intersex person doesn't classify themselves as "male" or "female."

*Love Languages*: In "The Five Love Languages," a book by Gary Chapman, the "love languages" include words of affirmation, quality time, physical touch, acts of service, and receiving gifts. You can take a test online that will tell you which of the love languages you "speak" the best (ranked by percentage), and this information can be used to improve your relationship. For example, if I like physical touch, but my partner like words of affirmation, then their love language may mean telling me how beautiful and sexy I am, and mine means I prefer giving my partner a back massage. When the other person knows where you stand, you can both understand each other's own way of expressing love.

*Polyamorous*: a.k.a. "poly" or "polyam" is a type of non-monogamous relationship dynamic. One or both partners may desire to be intimate with more than one person, while still maintaining the primary relationship, with their partner's informed consent. More people are leaning towards ethical non-monogamy (ENM) since it's becoming less taboo and more mainstream. There is discussion about replacing the term "poly" with "polyam," since "poly" can sometimes be used to refer to Polynesian people.

*Sir*: "Sir" is a BDSM term that two parties can choose to use in their relationship (either while playing in a scene or all the time, depending on the relationship). "Sir" is most often used in reference to or when addressing the dominant partner; however, sirs are typically gentler than a master. Other common terms for the dominant player include: Master/Mistress, Dom/Domme, or Top.

# 11

# NUDE BEACH MEETS THE DUNGEON

~It was his birthday, and each cop had a sexy alias name. Mine was "V" for Vixen, the sexy little wonder I had yet to uncover or fulfill the name's potential. It was as if Gabriel had seen my deepest self longing to come out before I did, or maybe I knew all along but had tamed her. This is where she started to shine and ground herself in the name. I welcomed her to try out a fun, sexy atmosphere that thrived on knowing yourself and your boundaries. Welcome to "Bikinis and Boardshorts (or Less)," the Nude Beach theme paying respect to the well-known beach and its vets. This is where the atmosphere of body-positivity meets kink and nightlife to the fullest. Welcome to the underground playground ... Welcome to self-discovery.~

*N*ude is a beach that is "clothing optional" in summer. It has a wonderful vibe—others take it upon themselves to make sure no one takes pictures or harasses anyone or gets in anyone else's space. We were born naked, so let us be naked by the sand without the prejudice of society projected onto it. Nude is a little hideaway, where you can get away. As soon as you get down the steps, through the magical old forest, an opening at the bottom, leading to the sandy beach, appears, and the heat and saltwater air hits your skin. The water is amazing for cooling off, and it goes in and out during the day, easing the cool's embrace. At sunset, we celebrate and give thanks to the sun—as if the sun was only meant for us that day—by dancing, drumming, and howling.

Our lovely Gabriel wanted to recreate this relaxed, peaceful, and respectful environment for people to chill inside during winter. He loved the vibe, the people, the sexiness, the fun, and the beautiful beach colors. Plus, he's into kink**, one reason why he decided to start little parties full of beach décor and beach wear, combined with dance music and the flare of nightlife. Needless to say, he was the king of the party front.

After throwing them for a few years, this particular party was for his birthday. Sexy cops dressed up and handed tickets out for a prize afterwards. We patrolled the place, spelling out "H-A-P-P-Y B-I-R-T-H-D-A-Y" on our asses for an on-stage surprise celebration, complete with cake. He became teary-eyed since his friends are family, and he holds us close to his heart.

Gabriel is OMG fit, tanned from selling freezies on the beach, with gorgeous flawless skin and a six-pack to match. He also has a freaking ass—man, I love a man with an ass. On top of all that, he is kind and sweet, and full of connection towards others. He would be there for you in your time of need, and lots of us would be there for him. Since this is the kind of people he attracts, people of integrity, warmth, and respect, Gabriel is gold … which leads me to wonder why he is single now … Hello, ladies! Looking for a gentleman who is fun and exciting? Sometimes, it's the raw jewels, the ones that aren't cut and shined, the ones that are humble and real, that we need to seek.

Now, back to the night that swept me away, the night I earned the nickname, stepped into it, owned it, and tumbled along the way …

We got to the club a little bit earlier to help set up with plastic badges, handcuffs, sexy tickets, and mini-markets. We also gave the "cops" a pep talk and went over what was required before they were off to patrol all the sexy fun, and we went upstairs to prepare the birthday boy's surprise in the hotel rooms. Saffron, Gabriel's GF at the time, was organizing this, and she was making it one to be remembered. Gabriel had no idea. There was a custom cake decorated in the theme from the party—3D people all dressed up on top. There were decorations galore, and then the music stopped so everyone in the club could sing him "Happy Birthday." He was in awe. When the song ended, we all spun around and showed off our asses to reveal H-A-P-P-Y B-I-R-T-H-D-A-Y spelled out. He laughed in amazement, and we took some pictures—with consent, of course—while he blew out his candles. He was speechless as he hugged and thanked each one of us, making sure we kept partying and being sexy. We handed out "too sexy to handle" tickets; one offence read, "Dancing too hot on the stripper pole while moving their hips seductively." The "offender" would get a surprise from Gabriel, who would be on stage with his hat on and a special freezie he had made with all organic ingredients. The freezies helped cool people down, and at the same time, ignited them to be oh so naughty throughout the night. The "cops" were also there in case anything went wrong or if something needed attention or safety needed to be enforced. We were the "consent crew," making sure the rules were enforced, even though everyone saw us as mostly welcoming newcomers and "enforcing" dancing. Let's just say I wore that outfit well!

Gabriel's parties always sold out because they were a blast. The vibes were killer, and people felt safe. Even though the culture was sex-positive** and body-positive*, there was no sex on the premises (SOP**), which was a rule we had to enforce since it required a special license. After dancing the night away and preparing for even more adventurous fun, the cops did a photoshoot together. Never a dull moment! The night flew by, but there was more to do. We had to make sure the club was shut down and everyone left.

My bestie, my Master**, and my forever friend went up to her room once more to collaborate about the night. She was tired and wanted to spend the rest of the night with her man, so Tristan and I moved on to our next adventure. Gabriel ended up continuing his birthday bash there as well. Our RV was already parked nearby; we had been preparing for a while for a long night. Being responsible, we made sure we had a place to crash so we wouldn't need to drive.

Our RV was amazing. Forty feet long, she had a queen size bed for us and a single for another. She was also remodeled and refinished with black shag carpet, marble floors, and a fresh interior. Just by looking at it, you wouldn't know how amazing it was inside because the outside still had its old retro paint job, giving away its age. It's what's inside that counts!

The party transitioned from sexy cops and lingerie to the RV and a bathing suit. I had heard there would be pools. I freshened up, getting ready to venture onward with Tristan. We were going to a Dungeon mansion party, where kink, fetish, and sex-positivity collided. This private party allowed for whatever your heart desired— SOP, music, food, drinks, sex swings, sex beds with black latex on top, condoms, wipes, you name it. Upon entering, you wouldn't know, however. The entrance was blackened out, and you were told to be discreet (quiet as a mouse!) and to not let anyone know where you were going or what you would be doing there. 'Twas a private ticket event where you would be signed in, your paid ticket scanned, and provided a wrist band before being allowed entry to explore.

Holy hotness, I explored, even got a little overloaded right from the get-go. There were entertainment bunnies in black latex, thong one-piece outfits with black bunny ear masks, heels, tails, and cuffs to match. Their job was to dance, play, and basically encourage bad behavior, but in a consensual way. With their not-so-real boobs out, the bunnies were all model-looking goddesses with slim, fit bodies and long, luscious hair—a few brunettes, a redhead, a blonde, one with black hair—done Victoria-secret style. They also greeted people as they walked in, making it all seem as if we were in a gentlemen's club.

The main floor was more chill—by that, I mean regular vanilla* type of foreplay—grinding, making out on top of each other, feeling about. This was where the food, drinks, and whatnot were, though more could be found in the different rooms. This mansion was huge, gorgeous, and beyond my expectations. Moving forward, there were stairs both up and down. We decided to go up. Along the way, we became more and more overwhelmed, seeing all the sensual, energetic people we knew, gesturing hellos, warm welcomes in passing. Everyone was either naked, partially naked, or wearing a get-up that turned heads. This was normal in my world, and how I loved it! This was what people dream about, watch movies for, or why erotic fiction is written. Needless to say, this was real, raw, and boy, was it charged with fun.

People there were dressed to impress, wearing barely-there lingerie, Mad Max, puppy/ kitten, low tails*, and so much more. There was latex bedding over everything to protect it from all kinds of fluids; two sex swings among the rooms; and as we circulated the top floor, going full circle, there were two (yes, not just one, but two!) saunas for people to decompress, relax, and dry off in. Moving through the crowd, I kept smiling in amazement.

One person was getting pounded on the sex swing while others fondled her, activating all the senses, hands, mouths, and other parts entangled in a big play**/sex scene of expression. In the other sex swing, a guy was getting sucked, poked, and devoured in pleasure. I looped around to make sure Tristan was following me since he was a tad slow for a tall, long-legged handsome guy. I kept grabbing his hand, all the while saying, "Omg look," or, "Wow," or even just giving a did-you-just-see-that look. He was giving a very boy-in-a-sandbox-wanting-to-play type of look. We ended our upstairs tour by stopping to play on a bench for a bit, taking in all the sounds. It got busier, and people started to get too close for my liking while I was going down on Tristan. He was almost getting fondled by someone else, shoved, and worse—touched without consent.

I asked to continue our journey, so we wandered downstairs. At the bottom of the mansion, there was a sauna and a pool table; a masked, shirtless firefighter with a six-pack was getting his ass kicked by a bunny cross-dresser who was strutting and flaunting her stuff like she'd been born in the killer spiked heels she had on. It looked as if they were playing doubles with a very well-dressed crossdresser in glittery heels and a fairy wearing pasties. She knocked a ball in a pocket and looked directly at me. Tristan tends to try to influence a lot of things without allowing me to just *be*. For instance, right then, he said, "You know you can go play with her if you like," as I locked eyes with the fairy. Frazzled by Tristan's comment, I blushed. I wanted Tristan. I loved these moments, but it seemed like, with our busy lives, they were becoming few and far between. It had been too long since we had just engulfed each other and spent time together. I said thanks and continued walking past the bar and pool table.

Where there was an opening outside, beautiful stone stairs led us up. It was a clear summer night out by the mountains, so a tad cool, but still not overly. Reaching the top, a heated pool awaited as well as a hot tub overflowing with naked bodies. It was pure magic how this all came together. It gave me ideas and then some. I wanted to wake up our dear friend who had gone to crash in our RV for a bit. We knew around a quarter of the people there, and there were a lot—in the hundreds. Needless to say, I had a hard time with all the energy spinning around. There were clashes, and some people were way too touchy flirty, if ya get what I mean.

There was one woman in particular that I recognized. She had red hair, bitch eyes, and a callous attitude. She teased and flirted with lots. I remember telling her off at a party—she was the one person in red—for not seeking consent before touching, and for grinding up and down on my man. I told her that was not consent, and she called me jealous, so then I told her off. Not my best moment. I said, "I don't have anything to be jealous of. He is my boyfriend, and that was just disrespect." She scowled and kept going till my boyfriend gave her a sexy ticket, after which I ripped his head off. Tristan, at that time, had no idea how to handle situations like that. Encountering her careless attitude, all those emotions came rushing back.

I tried to see if she remembered me, but she never even glimpsed my way beyond saying, "Hi, enjoying yourself?" I was nice and replied with a "yes," but nothing more. Tristan decided to carry on a conversation with her, with me in between. He apparently did not remember that incident either, or else he wouldn't have been so keen to chat more. He is very understanding about our boundaries**, or so I liked to think so.

I went over to the hot tub to soak my feet for a bit before Tristan and I wandered out through the gates back to our RV for some R 'n R. We needed it; I needed it. Our friend Brock was cuddling a pillow when I quickly got naked and started to wake him up per Tristan's suggestion. It was fun AND funny, especially since my other girlfriend was there for a bit to sit on him and make out with him while he mumbled awake and smiled, two naked women among him.

I kept thinking to myself, *This is better* … At big parties, where drugs, alcohol, and other things are astir, things can go awry or worse. Stuff goes sideways fast, lines get crossed, and other people are entwined … Usually, at afterparties, the later it gets, the more shit can go sideways. You can just sense it. You feel the energy, and boom, you know where the check-in point is, and you can ask, "Shall we go?"

In the RV, two other friends popped in, and we had our own mini-party, which was hilarious fun. Jokes were flying, people were massaging and groping each other. I was, of course, sucking off

Tristan, and I slid over to his friend's cock per Tristan's request. I sucked him off while Tristan watched. He loved it and wanted to fuck me hard after. It was his kink! And I had been the one to help him find it and remove the taboo for him. We loved exploring together …

Tristan took me from behind while I was still sucking his friend off, but the guy was only semi-hard, what with the drugs in his system and the booty he'd gotten earlier. He was done, and Tristan told him to try putting some "snow" power in the pee hole of his cock to bring him back. Tristan went first, and then he went from decent to roaring-thunder Viagra-style without the Viagra. He pushed my panties aside and pounded me on the single bed near the entrance while the others watched. Everyone was in awe …

I had been craving him all night. I wanted him, just *him* between my wet, juicy legs. My vulva was pulsing and swollen from the lust inspired by a whole night's tease, and when he took me, all that tension released, along with all the "Thank God" moans, high to low. The other guys watched with delight as my girlfriend rode my sleepy friend on the corner of the bed. He fingered her sleepily, while Tristan and I took up most of the single bed in the front. It felt amazing to share this space with people that I had dynamic, respectful relationships with. I was in my zone—sexy, sensual, and in the groove of sensation. Energy filled the room and so did the noises. The RV was where we were in sync, in sexual bliss, in ecstasy.

Suddenly, we heard a knock on the door, and we all stopped and covered up. It was Kyle's friend; he didn't know it, but we had been testing him to see if he could handle the party life. We said hi, and he asked to come in. He was drunk and sloppy, and I didn't want more people, especially ones I didn't know. Also, he had yelled over at this girl to tag along inside. I looked at Kyle and mouthed "no" (while saying, *Hell fucking no!* in my head). The night was over at the mansion, and others were out on the prowl, looking for more. Kyle went outside and chatted with his bud to basically try and ditch him. However, we ended up opening the door after deciding it was best to help him get home. He was being loud and stumbling around drunk. I was relieved when they left. We had clearly almost had a soon-to-be disaster on our hands and managed to side-step it.

We uncovered and continued, my girlfriend nipping at my nipples, telling me how nice they were and how hot it was to see me and Tristan fuck. Not just fuck, she said we "fuuuuucked" hard and shook the RV. He knew how to hit my spots deep. It was an especially lovely moment since my girlfriend knew I was a little self-conscious about my nipples and my boobs. My figure is tiny and so are my boobs to match. I always wanted a tad bigger. However, I always got the impression from others that they were a great size— enough to grab and not so big that they get in the way.

I was in awe. I liked the attention, the energy, the intimacy … The sleepy seductive friend moved his fingers towards me, helping Tristan out. All hands were on me, leading me into pure ecstasy once again. The sexual high was a pure rush. It seemed like I was in another world, one of true bliss, allowing the moment, the gentle swirls of my clitoral hood to get aroused and create more wetness for Tristan to keep pounding while my girlfriend continued to swirl her tongue on my nipples. I couldn't handle it anymore; I was vibrating, my muscles contracting with urge and release. I tensed and let out a moan of orgasmic pleasure. My sleepy friend, who wasn't so sleepy after all, said, "Thatta girl!" and Tristan was in awe, and my girlfriend just looked at me, her fingers moving from my clit over to her own. Her eyes said it all, as she used my wetness to lube her sore clit into more raging horny energy. She didn't last long in that atmosphere … while entwined, she came loud, saying, "Oh, yeah … oh, yeah," and, "More!" She closed her eyes, riding my friend's fingers while on top of him, to the end of her bliss. Tristan just petted me and watched with me. He had tried to cum, but it felt like he had a dozen times, and the drugs, as well as the tiredness, were making it hard to release fully.

Tristan and I quickly toppled towards the back to sleep, while the other two continued quietly or slept after her big, vibrating release and moan of, "OoooOOOOooo ..." The sun was rising, and we heard the birds starting their day. We had yet to sleep, and we needed to allow our bodies to rest up for another adventure. The Vixen needed to play ...

## The Lessons

Well, going to two parties in one night might have been overkill, but making a plan and having a place to be safe was gold! It is nice to have a spot to yourself, as well as one in which to crash just steps away. That RV became our "festie wagon." We bring it to parties to crash afterwards or to get ready, or to just have as a safe place to go back to. The RV has it all, and its cozy. Plus, we can have a few people over to chill or more.

The redhead—well, Tristan didn't know how to handle it, and she had really crossed the line into disrespect by groping and grinding all over him, wearing barely anything, at another party. Tristan and I chatted afterwards and realized it was his people-pleasing (not wanting to hurt people's feelings kind of thing). Trying to get out of a situation without hurting another was why he gave the redhead one of the sexy tickets. *Smooth, Tristan, smooth.* By not hurting *her*, you hurt me. At that time, I'm guessing he didn't even realize that's what he was doing. Trying to just get out of it *and* quickly, even if it may hurt another, Tristan had been under the influence of his avoidance attachment style*, which shows up in a tricky situation. We had discussions later about what went down and how to handle future events, plus what to say in situations where consent is given and when it's not given. Yes, this particular situation was a small thing, but these things have a way of leading to bigger things that can lead to bigger hurts. Best to *nip it in the bud*, i.e., get it out in the open and zone in on the opportunity for some positive attributes moving forward. At this party, Tristan hadn't recalled who she was till I mentioned it in the RV. Looking in his eyes, I could see the attention seeker. Glistening eyes always tell me he means something else. It is funny how well I can read him, and he is still learning about himself too.

This party had a lot, I mean *a lot*, of people. Some were from the previous party, others from other parties. For me, I was more interested in the layout and what it had to offer than in really taking part. I wasn't really into putting on a show where there was constant traffic. Now I know that isn't my thing. Tristan was up for anything, and I had moments, but I always need to be comfortable or else it really isn't fun, and it shows in my body language and overall energy. Ask yourself where your comfort level is; what's ok versus what's not ok, and what kind of scenes** you are willing to partake in. These are great questions to explore and see what fits. You may have things you want to try. I wouldn't have thought I was gonna put on a show in the RV, or achieve pure bliss like that, but man, oh man, was that fun! Five-star rating for RV fun, will come back, LOL!

Some things to consider: Do you know your limits? Do you know your partner's limits? Do you have safe words** or cues to check in, or rather, both "check out" to go somewhere and chat? What is comfortable versus uncomfortable in the moment? Anything you want to try? What are both of your intentions, if any, for the night? Is it ok to play or touch? Is there an end time? Remember to take breaks and hydrate.

This was the night "The Vixen" was born, where the name started to take shape …

## Glossary

*Attachment Styles*: There are four main attachment styles, which are ingrained into you basically from birth to 18 months. The first style is secure; just like it sounds, you can self-sooth, count on your caregiver to be there, and so forth. The second is an anxious attachment style, which is basically a fear of being alone. It can look like people-pleasing, low self-esteem, validation seeking, and a need to be in the know. The third is an avoidance or dismissive attachment style; the person is independent, distant, ambivalent, and basically uncaring if needed in a situation. This style includes a fear of intimacy, vulnerability, and commitment. The fourth is a fearful or ambivalent attachment style, which is characterized by avoidance, insecurity, poor boundaries, hot/cold personality, and—you guessed it—runs on fear. These styles were introduced by Bowlby and further developed by Ainsworth in the field of Behavioral Psychology.

*Body-Positivity*: An attitude or approach in which people are free to express themselves in how they dress; free to be any shape, size, gender, orientation; free from judgment and discrimination; essentially, your body, your choice; absolutely no shaming.

*Low Tails*: This accessory usually indicates that a person is wearing a butt plug with a tail attached.

*Vanilla*: This term refers to people who are monogamous, or those who aren't familiar with kink, fetish, or lifestyle worlds. "Vanilla" could also be used for people who are new to the scene.

# 12

# NIGHT OF THE RACCOON

~He was what the universe was waiting for me to accept into my life, right after I had closed the book on a chapter only two weeks prior. He caught me off guard; he knew my people, was connected, and in the scene I am in. He was himself growing and exploring, something I noted, and I was down to see what he was exploring too. I wanted to know him, truly know him— every hurt, successes, ups, downs, and scars. I wanted to know all about his passions, his visions, his quiet moments. I wanted to nuzzle into his welcoming arms and never leave and just lie with him on a beach and adventure at night. I wanted to explore the world and our bodies. Longing for a certain person I felt intensely about so instantly scared me. He turned my world upside down in a good way. His eyes turned from blue to green depending on the environment and situation, like a chameleon. His energy was powerful, making my femininity shine even more. He worked hard and played hard, and I couldn't wait to be part of it.~

The meet ...

*M* y eyes widened at the name "Garden of Eve" on his tongue, and suddenly, I could hear my heart race. He started chatting about this club I knew so well, describing the scene to me without realizing I already knew. I wanted more; I wanted to hear how he described the play** at the club with its loads of stories and more to come, places that I had yet to see and to conquer. I looked into his eyes and saw the moment the conversation eased, like he didn't want to give away too much, didn't want to fully express what the club was exclusively known for. I assumed he was being cautious when he momentarily quieted his voice while describing some aspects of the place and turned to me to ask if I had been. I smiled and said, "Ahhh ... you are talking about Garden of Eve." Shocked, he said, "Yeah ... How do YOU know about Garden of Eve?" with a smirk. Without thought, without judgment, and without momentary weakness, I said, "Oh, I know about Garden of Eve. I know Garden of Eve very well." His only reply was a taken-aback look, and it was clear he wanted to know more.

We connected instantly without knowing fully why. His presence took me by surprise, but I also felt like I just *knew* him. He and I chatted as the night progressed into a Kava ceremony* and more connecting. I wanted to be close to him, wanted to know more about why I wanted such a thing too. I didn't want to hold back; I could tell he had an interesting past as his genuine self indicated as much. He was mysterious, and he amazed me. He got closer as the night continued; I flirted without knowing where it would take me. He had caught something of mine that I'd been holding on to for so long, something that had been stitched up and mended time and time again.

I danced the night away, moving in my flowy black dress with its very well-placed V-neck mesh that plunged to my waistline. I caught his smile as he looked at me through the glass from outside while I talked to the chief about life, relationships, ceremonies, and presence. I could feel him—his warmth, his touch, his on-going inquiry as to who I might be. I turned from my conversation and smiled at him, knowing full well that he would be looking right at me. I blew a kiss, winked, and laughed, and he gave me such warmth and acceptance, gleaming back at me from within.

I only carried on the conversation with the chief a little longer before going back inside, pulled in by the magnetic sexual polarity* we had. We carried on where we had left off. He said, "I think your boyfriend would mind if you went to Garden of Eve with me." I smiled and said, "What boyfriend?" We took in the moment, and in that moment, we both knew we wanted so much more than fun; we had a connection, we had polarity, and we were interested in finding out more.

We talked most of the night and stared into each other's eyes while venturing around in each other's worlds. He was an entrepreneur at heart and played well at it: direct, focused, driven, and well-maintained. He knew he could succeed, and so he did; the power of intention was on his side and so was the law of attraction. This was not only true in his life but also in mine. As recently as two weeks ago, I was still holding on to nothingness and giving my energy when it was no longer healthy. I had cut ties and pushed forward so a new light could shine and guide me towards new beginnings. I'd written out my ideal man just weeks before and reading it again had helped me set my intentions regarding who I wanted to attract into my life.

After letting the night take me away in a flirtation spiral, I said goodnight, gave him a leaping hug and kissed him goodnight. He asked me to stay, just to sleep even. I hesitated and said I had promised my friend that I would catch up with him, and so I hustled downstairs. Giggly with excitement, I longed to stay with him some more, but I denied myself the satisfaction as I was coming to understand that what we had was what I thought it was.

I talked with my friend till the wee hours of the morning and crashed at dawn … among other things. In the morning, I awoke excited and nervous to catch up with my new friend—or soon-to-be lover—for a surprise cuddle session. To my surprise, the couch was empty, the cushions realigned, the blankets and pillows folded and neatly piled on top of each other. My heart sank and then I knew he was a tad different, but I wasn't going to jump to conclusions. I sat, looking outside the window at the beautiful morning that came. Smiling, I got up and looked around. His bear claw necklace had been left behind. I thought it could be a great excuse to see him again, so I texted him to let him know he'd left his necklace there and asked, "Where did you go off to so early?" His necklace had been made by a chief that was called to make them for people who had participated in an Ayahuasca ceremony*. He texted back, telling me to keep it till we saw each other again. Maybe at Garden of Eve for Halloween? I replied with a sly grin, "You're on."


Our Halloween went from just us to seven in total: one raccoon, four cats, a doctor, and a tennis player. None had been to Garden of Eve before except Tristan and I this was bound to be an adventure and a half as we both didn't know each other very well, and I also only had a little connection with everyone in the car. After introductions, the nervousness could be felt in this car full of unexplored individuals.

Turning up the tunes and not knowing what to expect, I knew everyone else had no idea what the club was even about. Tom asked about the club, and me and Tristan just looked at each other, beaming about what to expect. He rubbed my leg, keeping his big, warm hands on me as I blushed like a little schoolgirl.

Once there, everyone knew Tristan and me. We both said hi to our individual groups and introduced our party with big smiles on deck. We gave a tour, the newbies signed a waiver, and we all did a little photoshoot so we would have a memory of that night before we all got displaced.

As the night progressed, Tristan and I grew apart. He was off dancing with Britney and making out with her. I didn't understand nor did I want conflict, so I passed it off as he just did this with everyone and that I was no one special after all. Once I got that through my head, I headed out to the bar to say hi to everyone and revive my parched throat with some aqua times dose. Back on the dance floor, I wandered over to Tom to dance and make out, getting my sexy on and rubbing up against his semi-erect cock, thinking I could pop that boy up if I wanted to. Seeing as Tristan had been nowhere in sight for a long time now, I asked Tom if he had seen upstairs yet. He nudged me to show him, and as we slid our way, we ran into more creatures of the night we knew and stopped to chat. While chatting, Tom was pulled away by two ladies who were fondling him all over and caressing him, so he continued upstairs with them. I moved to his side to say hi, and the other girl had no interest in having fun with me, what with her black hair, polished makeup, and batty fake lashes that rolled with her eyes in disgust at the thought of conversing with me. I stepped back and whispered to Tom to have fun as he wanted to have fun with all three. I couldn't do that, not with a girl who acted like that.

I moved past them and nodded a go-ahead for him and the other two to mosey on up. He swung around and hunched his shoulders, his hands up at me as if wanting me to help him. The girls were touching him and circling around his body as if he was their new bait and marking him as such. Laughing, I swayed over to the dance floor, letting the music take me away with it. I closed my eyes to the movement and light that filled the dark space for the throbbing dancing crowd.

Moving past my insecurities until they were absent, I started dancing with the other kittens from our crew. The blonde was a little vanilla; the bigger one wanted to play, and by play, she meant kissing and licking along my boob line and finally just pulling my top down to expose my hard nipples. My tits were plump—a solid B—but hers were big, as in DD and swinging out for more exposure. She nibbled and kissed as she laughed at how open I was. I winked at her in agreement, and we started making out, diving deep into each other while the skinny Asian cat played with her pussy, trying to wedge in for more play time.

I plotted back after the bigger one started to touch and fondle my thighs, leading up to my already longing moist core, which was only really longing for one. I didn't hesitate nor pull away from her eager hands; I moved down on her, dancing and touching her on my way up from the dance floor. I kissed her pussy as I eyed her from in between her legs. She screamed at me and said, "Bitch, you got sass." I smiled back at her and nuzzled into her kahoonas while she wiggled me into them more. I wanted to ask her for more play as well; I craved more and couldn't handle myself any longer.

As the Asian kitty pried in between us and forced her tongue down my throat, I pulled back. I was taken aback by her gesture and aggression as only moments ago, she had been by herself, barely dancing with a resting bitch face plastered on. I hadn't felt like approaching her at that point in time, but now—holy smack, 180 switch—she was dancing, fondling, and pushing through for aggressive kissing that I couldn't stand. Her tongue was hard as rock and pegging my mouth as if she were fucking it. I pulled her hair back, thinking, *No girl does that to me*, and started aggressively kissing her back, taking her as she moaned and let me in. She was a bad kisser from the start and by putting myself in the aggressor position, I could slip away towards Tristan, who had finally showed up. I left for more water, and I saw his eyes gleam over at me, wondering why I had gone.

I smiled, thinking this night was going be interesting. At least now I knew that he wasn't as interested as I'd thought. I came back to the dance floor and danced away to the brilliant DJ blaring awesome tunes, and soon realized that Tristan had been with Britney the whole time. I now understood my place and started dancing with him. As he got closer, he whispered in my ear to ask if I wanted to check upstairs, and I nodded. We then swung around to get everyone else before proceeding upstairs.

We all pushed our way upstairs; Tristan now looked more like a veterinarian with a raccoon and four cats following him upstairs. Hearing the moans and seeing the sights of naked bliss, the pussy cats called up, "Wow, orgy." I smiled at the sights. Nowhere was open so we had to continue further up the stairs, climbing past an orgy bed full of arms and legs, where beginnings and ends were unknown at this point. My favorite room with the St. Andrew's cross** "X" was coming up and where we would stop; the smaller room inside that room was busy, but we stayed, and the rest followed.

Tristan sat down and watched the cats dance together and touch me in the process, our arms and hands swaying with the beat as our legs were all intertwined in ecstasy while we made out with each other. When I opened my eyes, I saw that Britney was the last one I had kissed. I slowly moved away and started dancing with Tristan, bumping and grinding my butt into his crotch. I gave him permission to take me since I had been the one longing for him all this time. He turned me around and kissed me passionately.

I didn't know what to expect as I had thought he wasn't into me as much as I'd hoped, but then he turned me towards the bench and I pounced on top of him, rubbing against him, getting hot and bothered. I couldn't help myself and our surroundings slowly stopped mattering as much. The three other girls were still making out, and he slipped his hands down to see how wet I truly was. I was soaked, wanting him, and his sex. I pressed my wet pussy against his hand as he was eager to push my panties aside. He unbuckled his belt, unzipped and grabbed my round ass towards him, gliding me against his erect cock. I felt it throbbing for me and I for it. Breathing heavy, I whispered, "I want you." He pushed me up, holding me, as I grabbed on and he moved his way towards the wall, pressing me up against it. I loved it—his dominance, his masculine energy, his taste, and his touch. I was in pure motion, closing my eyes to be present to the sensations of the moment; to let myself release; to let go and let him take me, but I still felt a slight resistance, not knowing what he thought. I didn't want to be just an object, just another girl. I wanted more than that, something real. He pushed harder into me, and I felt high on life itself.

The girls trickled away, leaving us as we moved back to the bench to fully engage each other. He slowly tipped me as I hadn't had a throbbing thick cock for a while, and even though I was wet, I needed the tender touch and slow bliss of his gentle nature. I straddled him on the bench and started passionately kissing him, so there was no question what I wanted. I pushed my panties aside. Once in, I trembled at the sensation of him; he felt amazing. His dick wasn't too big in length, so as not to hurt me, and it was thick enough to make me squirm … *Perfect,* I thought. I knew we would get along and so did our privates. He started pressing me in more; it hurt a bit, only momentarily as it had been a while since I had experienced such beauty.

I wanted him. I wanted his skin touching mine. My animal started to come out in a natural flow, and I grabbed him, pressing into every kiss, every movement and pumping into him, propping my hand on the red wall for stability and placing my other hand on the backside of his head. He switched from grabbing my ass with both hands to push deeper into me to supporting my back and my ass at the same time. I moaned, and he loved it. We were heated and going into each other—looking, kissing, fondling, and pressing our foreheads together as the sweat created a slippery layer for us while we panted.

Britney and the cats came into the room while we were fucking to ask us where the other vanilla cat had gone, with no consideration for what we were doing. She paused, looked at us momentarily and said, "Ok, sorry for the interruption." We shrugged and went back to kissing. Shortly after, we were parched and needed water. We grabbed a glass from just outside the door (this club had thought this out) and eyed each other before proceeding.

He led me into the next room, bypassing the orgy bed to the sex swing. Surprisingly, no one was there. "Oh, look at that," he said with a half-grin. I plopped myself up on it without a struggle

(J/k, I wedged my way on it like a beached whale, half-tired and trembling from satisfaction). He swung me in to kiss me and kissed me down there as well. The swing had been adjusted just right for us. As he started swinging me into place, Bre poked her head in with her boyfriend, screeching, "Oh, crap! How long are you gonna be?" I replied, "Sorry, hun, just got here." She smirked, saying it was her favorite spot. I told her my favorite spot was taken. Meanwhile, Tristan was looking at me with an *ok, let's carry on* kind of look as he was already inside me. I laughed and said *sorry*. I asked Bre to leave the door open with a wink and a smile. She smiled, laughed, and went on her merry way.

Tristan looked at me and kissed me. The room was tiny, and the swing was fun and easy to use, but I wanted the weight of our bodies pressing on us. He pounded me, using the swing to push me into him as I held on for dear life. It was fun, but he was growing tired, so onward we went … We didn't have to look for long, plopping down on the bench just out front of that room, which overlooked the dance floor. I sat on top, threw my legs around him and rode him, leaning back, then forward again, grabbing his sweat-beaded face to kiss. I was sweating as well—more like *drenched*. Tristan fingered me in place as I rode, breathed, and moaned, closing my eyes and grabbing him close as I came. I trembled and kissed him as our hot breath was on each other's faces.

Getting up, our legs were tired and weak. We looked around, soon realizing we were missing clothes. I said, "This is the fun part." He said, "What's that?" I said, "The scavenger hunt!" He laughed as we backtracked to find his pants behind us, his belt and my costume ears in the sex-swing room, and his shirt in the very first room we were in. We looked at each other and smiled, exhausted but ready to go downstairs to dance and recoup. Downing water after water, we once more made the trek to the dance floor. We swayed and danced a little longer, made out with the girls, touching, fondling. Before I knew it, I was sandwiched between the girls, getting played with and loving it as Tristan watched, smiling.

Hungry, we all left for pizza. All dressed in scantily clad wear—or mostly just me—we got looks. We were all still fondling each other too. Britney and Tristan made their way into the pizza place while me and Tom waited and exchanged stories.

Once the afterparty was announced, the rest of the girls left, but me and the guys pushed forward to an EAST house party. Inside, I saw Tiffany and slapped her ass instantly while everyone around waited to see if we actually knew each other. She swung around and jumped on me, and I introduced her to the guys while she was still mounted on me. She introduced me to her boy-toy and sat down while we fondled each other's asses in the process and kissed. Tristan and Tom looked on with surprise and off we went for a tour of the place. I kissed who I knew along the way. Downstairs, there was a separate kitchen, a room lit with candles and a sex bed; the other room was for shows with its spank bench and a couch for viewing.

Once back upstairs, Tiffany grabbed me so we could have fun with her boy. Her boy liked to ass-worship, so he was set up at the base of the sex bench to best nuzzle his face in Tiffany's ass. She was bent forward, telling me to get my ass on the other side of the bench because she wanted to taste me. I wasn't going to say no, and I wasn't afraid of putting on a show; I loved it. I sat up on the bench and almost fell over because she was getting pushed by her boy on the other end and shoving her face into my pussy. I didn't mind at all, but my back could hardly support me. One of the onlookers noticed and suggested holding me; he wouldn't fondle me unless I asked. I agreed—and thank God I did—it was bliss-in-motion. Tiffany knew my spots and her moans vibrated onto my clit as I pressed backwards, gripping onto my holder as he petted me cautiously. I acknowledged his presence and his movements, letting him know how I felt. I said, "Wow, that actually feels really good!" with a surprised look. (Not sure why I had a surprised look on.)

After a little while, we all switched and I was on the bottom, getting ass-worshiped (I found it amusing that I had never experienced this before either). I let him wriggle his face into my ass, not knowing what was to come or what to expect. I wanted to loosen up and *wow*, did I ever. I was able to go down on Tiffany, and the crowd was amazed at how well I knew her body. They commented on just that. I realized I could read her, licking and tickling her clit in so many ways, making her moan and shake. She would bite her lip and make the best sounds as her legs shook with pleasure and she pat my head … While she patted me, I looked up at her in surprise and said, "Wait, did you just pat me like a 'good dog'?" She started laughing and so did I. The onlookers in the room laughed too.

I shook my head and moved on to tasting her after grabbing an ice cube. She jumped, and I said, "That's what you get for patting my head." We both smiled and carried on. They boy took a break and just watched a bit as me and Tiffany were having fun just by ourselves. She wanted more ass-worship as that was her favorite; it drove her crazy. We switched up the train once more, all the while grabbing ice cubes and water to freshen up a bit. We went at it till my back couldn't handle it anymore. When we stopped, we got comments from the crowd that had formed; they told us how hot we were and thanked us for the performance. We smiled, knowing it was true as Tiffany and I had the best view of all.

While making our way back upstairs, my friend Scotty grabbed me to go see the "ballroom." I was thinking it was a dance room until we got to the top and he threw me in a room upstairs that was full of balls, like a ball pit. I laughed hysterically at how amazing it was, and sooo comfy. Eight of us played in the ball pit, throwing balls at each other. Then we tried to hit the light with them. (I wasn't sure why this was so entertaining. Was I high?) Tristan came up with a half-surprised look on his face, knowing full well how things like this end up. Then Tiffany and the boy piled in.

I told Tristan it was great because you don't know what's going on underneath the balls, and I looked him up and down, already neck deep. We started smirking and fondling, and everyone started to fade away except the four of us. Getting fingered in a ball pit with Tiffany saying, "No fair, I can't see!" was the only downside.

The balls were forgiving but everywhere. I climbed on top of Tristan and played with Tiffany's ass, all the while kissing Tristan. What an amazing night … I threw balls out from in between us so he could penetrate me more, but it was time to move on at that point.

While riding the boy, still immersed in balls, Tiffany looked at us. "After-after party?"

Tristan and I looked at each other and grinned, ready for more …

Once at the boy's place, we opened the door to a heat wave. There was a fireplace and a cat that ran around like a spaz. I ran over to the fireplace right away, happy for the comfort. The night wasn't over yet, but my back was sore from before. Tristan lay next to me as we undressed and cuddled naked. I just wanted that moment to stay forever; it was warm and passionate. Naked cuddles are the best. I felt like the luckiest woman. Tiffany and the boy had a mini ass-worship session in the other room while we lay in front of the fireplace, basking in each other's energy and presence.

The boy came back out for a drink and Tristan got up to join him on the couch, leaving me naked and exposed. Tiffany took the opportunity to pounce, and I laughed when she said, "Well, isn't that convenient?" I smiled at her and reminded her about my back before she just spread my legs and pleasured me right in front of the two on the couch. I loved it; she licked, fondled, and played around. It was great with her tongue ring, a little round surprise. She fingered me in the process. I was getting aroused, moaning and squirming a little. Tiffany's boy got turned on, so she went into the bedroom, asking him to follow.

Tristan lay where Tiffany had been and started finishing what she had started, making me move and arch like no other. I gasped for air, trying hard not to cum right away. I wanted the feeling to last. Then Tristan pulled me up to go join Tiffany and the boy in the room so we could play side by side with them, mimicking their every move. Well, almost. Tiffany loved ass-worship, and I just loved getting pounded from behind. It was easy on my back, and I could feel him more. I liked it hard, grabbing the sheets and squeezing my eyes shut at the sensual feelings that arose. Tiffany was in the same position. I kissed her lying down, panting hard and telling Tristan, "She really likes what you're doing." His reply was a simple "good" with a sly smirk. It was the boy's first side-by-side play and sex party. And everything felt amazing. Tristan came in a cup nearby and I made my way back to the fireplace. I looked at my rug-burned knees and felt my sore back, but I didn't care as the evening was yumminess and the fire eased it all.

After refueling with water and a granola bar, I looked at the time and started searching for my raccoon ears and my underwear. I found the ears across the room and my underwear was misplaced, probably because of that crazy cat that was going all Miss Spaztastic. She had been trying to steal my ears before so she must have stolen my underwear now. Ah-ha! They were on the floor near the side table. Looking at the time and realizing it was now 8 am, Tristan was already late for his meeting. Before we hustled out, I kissed Tiffany goodbye while she was giving head to the boy. She was sad to see me leave, but she was busy, and we had to rush, despite our total bliss and sex exhaustion … We said goodbye with a starry-eyed kiss in the quiet of the morning, brisk mist on our faces. He let go of my hand and rushed away, dialing in for his meeting …

## The Lessons

First off, yes, you guessed it: I should have asked what Tristan's intentions were with me from the start. Him asking me to go to Garden of Eve for Halloween made a nice ASS-umption outta me. I thought it was—you guessed it—a date. My confusion and rough knowledge of the facts presented made it very hard for me to decipher his intentions. Then he made out with me, then my girlfriend … umm, this confused me even more. However, I still wouldn't change what I did as the confusion didn't affect my night or change my mood. I just let me be me. And by doing so, I had one hell of a night.

Also, make sure to keep your clothes with you wherever you go; you never know when you might lose your wallet or even your underwear to someone or some crazy cat. Just be cautious—a scavenger hunt while navigating around naked, sex-crazed people can be pretty hilarious. It is a lot easier to have your clothes with ya at all times. Plus, losing my cute costume ears would have made for a sad raccoon.

When you get dragged downstairs by your girlfriend to play, bring the rest of your crew to watch or at least let them know. I wasn't thinking; I should have just dragged the rest of us along as well because hey, who doesn't like putting on a show and being in the sexually energetic train flow?

When dropping off friends to their cars, make sure to double check with them, as in say: "HEY, it's a Saturday, and there might be roadblocks. You sure you don't want to just come and crash where we are going?" That night, one of the girls got hit with a roadblock and got her license taken away and her car impounded as well. #roadsense. Just look out for each other. We tried by saying, "You good?" but forgot to remind her it was Saturday—and a holiday at that. And worse, she was going over a bridge. But it's true that you can only do so much.

Going in for a threesome and then turning it down—this happened that night. There was going to be a guy and three girls, but I was smart ... S-M-A-R-T. All parties involved were not 100% and that made it awkward. Once I felt that, I was out. No *if, ands, or buts*. Sex/play is a tricky thing, and a solid "Fuck yes" is a must. A solid "FUCK YEAH!" It's like tea—you don't shove tea down someone's throat if they don't want it. NO, you don't!

Lastly, when there is a cat that likes your ears, tail, and underwear, HIDE THEM. Or else you will be on a hunt for your clothes yet again since that crazy cat will have taken them and you'll be tired, sore, and not wanting to play this game at 8:00 am so you can hurry home and your already-late man can get to his meeting.

# Glossary

*Ayahuasca Ceremony:* An ancient ceremony in Peru where you drink a brewed aya plant that activates DMT in your body (which is only there when you are born and dying, hence why some have a "rebirthing" experience). This should only be done by an indigenous shaman who knows the ancient ways of his culture. You will also need to pre-screen to make sure you do not do this if you have any medical conditions or are on any medication or drugs. The mother plant medicine is said to help guide you towards your growth, move you through blocks, and enlighten your understanding of the universe. It has been used to help people who have anxiety, depression, PTSD, etc. Do your research beforehand as well.

*Kava Ceremony:* An ancient ceremony where you sit in a circle in front of the leader or group facilitator, and you communicate your intentions and gratitude and all drink at once (this is how we did it). Kava root is known for its power to connect to the soul and for promoting relaxation naturally. It can make your tongue tingle a bit.

*Sexual Polarity:* Occurs when masculine and feminine dynamics are in sync with each other in perfect harmony or pleasure. Energy entwines the two as if nothing else matters—no thoughts, only the senses, pleasure, and oneness. David Deida says in his book *Intimate Communion*, "Sexual polarity—the magnetic pull or repulsion between the Masculine and Feminine—affects all our lives."

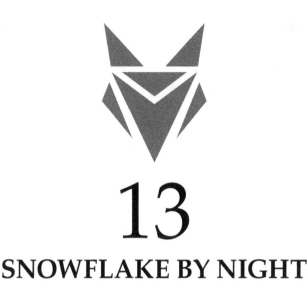

# 13
## SNOWFLAKE BY NIGHT

~Newly invited and wanting more … Forever drawn to your everlasting presence, my heart throbs and races … Thoughts of you—aching, pulsing, running through my veins—no hesitation, no doubt. My mind can't decipher the emotional eruption of your effect on me. You forever will affect my heart even when my mind has no understanding. You moved me, mirrored me, and touched my soul … ~

*K*nowing me, I was craving more, my intentions running in line with the universe itself. I smiled as I made my costume. I still had white fur from a previous party ("James," I said, chuckling). I sewed white fur shoulder pads to my bra, made a white fur headpiece (almost like an angel), and put on white lingerie to match, complete with white stockings and white fur boots. I was a sexy little snowflake.

Fifteen of us met up at Garden of Eve. We were all new to the scene except three of us, two of which were Tristan and me. The night ended with three newly-made couples (yes, I'm that good). When making a space for exploration and adventure in a safe, exciting environment with a solid group, things are bound to happen … as they always do when I am involved …

I was concerned when I didn't hear back from Tristan. He wasn't waiting for me outside the club, so I was getting nervous and self-conscious … But why? I got triggered back to the first party we'd gone to. He had knowingly made out with my friend, off doing who knows what. *Is he doing the same thing tonight? Is what we have all in my head?* I thought I was losing it, so I laughed at myself—at my ego for going on a tangent and giving meaning to something that hadn't even happened (Crazy, RIGHT?!).

I gathered everyone (They all looked sexy as hell), and they looked around nervously because they hadn't been there before. I chuckled and away we went. Once inside, I undressed near the lockers to the simple stares (plus a "wow" followed by a "hot damn") of everyone filling out the forms together. I smiled and told them about the video they needed to watch and the most important rules to pay attention to, all while directing them like a flight attendant in my scantily clad white. As I was talking, I kept getting smirks and comments like: "Wait, say that again. I can't concentrate when you're not wearing … well …" That helped boost my ego a tad and gave me more self-confidence, considering my phone still had zero messages on it. I ignored it. Once everyone was done, I told them to proceed to the back for a tour to be led by Cupid Amanda with wings (She waved).

I continued with Clair for a private tour because she was the more nervous of the bunch, and she had been ready before everyone else. We pushed forward, and there was Tristan with a nervous-looking Candice. I didn't know what to think of her reaction to seeing me; it seemed like she was hiding something, but I trusted my gut and didn't let it ruin anything. I gave Tristan a half-kiss-hug and joined Clair for her tour and to chat with her more about

"Nervous Nancy" jitters. After telling her about the place and the rooms, she thanked me for the private viewing, and I could feel her tension release a bit. I had also told her not to expect anything since she would not be expected to do anything either.

Once we were downstairs again, we saw that everyone was still on the tour, so I went back to the table that was reserved for us and sat to chat with the ladies. Tristan got up and followed me while I went to get a drink. He motioned for me to move back to chat; there was a slight tension between Candice and Clair. I said, "Roger," and headed back to the table, plopping myself in between them. I carried the conversation, all the while thinking that I wasn't the only one who felt this tension. Candice said something about Clair that I didn't like, but I couldn't understand why, so I wanted to give her the benefit of the doubt and try to get to know her.

We chatted about pole dancing since I had just bought a pole hours earlier (Yeah, I did, and I love it!). The music was great as always, with great vibes. We headed to the dance floor, and I could see that Candice had a thing for Tristan. This made me uneasy. When I looked at her looking at Tristan, she would look away. *Not a good sign*, I thought. I looked back at him, and he was smiling back at her. I asked him what that was about. He shook his head and said, "Nothing." Again, my nerves spiked, and I didn't like it. I went to go get everyone and to make sure everything was going smoothly.

When I got back, Candice was dancing with Tristan, and when they saw me, they both scattered. She lowered her eyes in submission as if we were in the animal kingdom and I was the alpha. I looked around and shook my head, knowing what that was, but I wasn't going to dive into it now. I wanted to party and dance the night away with no worries.

After a quick photo session with naughty Santa (oh yeah, this was a Christmas party if you didn't get that already, complete with bad elves at play). Tristan and I couldn't handle ourselves after that naughty shoot, and we wanted our time together. We hurried up to floor three and ripped off our clothes in a moment of lust, seduction, and longing infatuation. Eyeing each other, we kissed passionately. I didn't want to think about anything that had happened prior, so I let my thirst take control of my body and mind.

As I was sucking him off, we heard another tour coming through. I downed him, all of him, making my eyes water with his thickness and stern shaft. I handled it well considering my gag reflex. I used the corkscrew*, a lovely technique I had picked up and added a twist of my own—I like to use my hands and my mouth combined. Boy, did it drive him wild. He pushed the door closed and said, "I don't want to scare the newcomers off … yet." I smiled. His mind always went to the gutter. His language matched mine, and I loved it. He couldn't handle it anymore, so he pushed me down on the bed in the red room, propped my legs against the wall for more leverage, and pounded me. I had to move back a bit as his throbbing cock was too big to handle at that exact moment. But he was able to slide in once my wet pussy lips had a taste. My heart throbbing, I screamed with pleasure … Moaning and scratching for more, I trembled (I tend to do this a lot before I cum). Trembling and gasping for air, I released and threw my hands down. He kissed me gently. Panting, we were both sweaty.

I smiled at his sweet side. He had a calming effect, a grounding notion, and we had sexual polarity**. Still inside me, he slowly glided out, and we got dressed, smiling in elegant bliss at the ravishing behavior we had just indulged in (in my favorite room, of course). We headed back to the dance floor before time took us in its grasp. Everyone was in full dance mode and enjoying the night. We both smiled; no one had noticed our little getaway, even though we were both sweaty and beaming light. We moved towards a couple and kissed them under the candy-cane mistletoe attached to their heads. We all enjoyed each other's juiciness. The music took me in its grasp and away I went, naughty little snowflake falling low to the floor like nobody's business.

We moved towards a sexy couple that Tristan knew (swinging away), and then we all left to go once more upstairs … I was actually a little uncomfortable since Tristan and I had not had that talk yet, let alone played with others. In the room, he started kissing and fondling her … like I'd never asked. I looked puzzled about what was to come of this. He said, "Surprise …" It was as if he thought I wanted this, as if he knew me already, but it was far from what I wanted. I kept looking at Tristan, hoping he would look at me as he went to kiss her, but it never happened … and that's when I felt it … the disconnect. The "only sex" act and nothing more. Her top was still on and so was mine, and they both grabbed condoms. I told myself to speak up, yet I couldn't make my voice heard, not even a peep. *I will talk to him after so as not to kill the mood,* I thought. I wouldn't stop something that had already begun. My trust was in him and only him or else I wouldn't be doing what I was doing. I knew he had played with them before. They were a hot couple—fit, sexy, gorgeous. They were married swingers** who were picky (*Thank God*, I thought). My energy and strength were my own and not to disperse … All I wanted was a sign that he and I were still connected. It never came, even at the end.

While he was fucking her missionary, the other guy was fucking me missionary. I was numb … looking for any sign, anything … hoping he would see my fear or my uncertainty. I never mentioned anything at that moment. I couldn't. I was stuck, mute and still. As they finished, I put on a smile, got dressed quickly, and left to the washroom to freshen up. I let out a tear of pain and disbelief over what had happened. I had never felt that way before, had never been sexually numb to the point of shock and inability. I looked in the mirror and splashed water on my face before going into a stall to reconnect with myself and to try and understand what happened to me. But I couldn't, and this was not the time. I wanted the night to finish … I swept my situation under the rug and pretended it hadn't happened. I avoided it and avoided the hot couple. I couldn't face my inner pain yet or my turmoil and confusion.

We preceded downstairs to dance more and saw our friends all around the pole, dancing. The two dancers were epic, exotic, and in tune with themselves and their desires. They moved together, in sync with the music, spinning on the pole, around and below. Following each other, their energy flowed and more. I wanted to see more from them, so I asked if they had gone upstairs yet. They said no ... I suggested showing them if they were interested ... No need for play**, of course, but I told them I would love to see them play. They looked at each other with questioning eyes, and the woman leaned over to tell me that this was the first time they had danced together. All I could muster up was, "Wow ... such chemistry in the way you guys move together ... Took my breath away." It literally did. You had to be there.

They agreed to see the upstairs, and I motioned for Tristan to join. We proceeded to go upstairs and that was when I decided to show them around. We went to the room that I call my fav (once more) ... red lit and small ... for less clothes. I walked them in, closed the door, and my coaching began ...

I let them know the rules, that they were allowed to stop at any time, and yes, they wanted to come upstairs too. I told them they could say no to anything and that we were just here to support. Tristan and I started to party, and then Trevor and Lila started. This was their first time being intimate, and wow! So hot. They were both unbelievably hot ... passionate and vibrating.

We continued, and I directed (one of my kinks**). This was my man's first guy-on-guy kiss ... Took him by surprise. It was kinda funny to see him caught off guard. I was all into the woman by my side, and then I told Trevor it was his turn. He played with Lila as I kissed her, and Tristan went down on me, touching my crevices and tickling my baby hairs with his tongue, as if he knew my body already. I bit my lip in sensational overload. Pleased with myself, I wanted him, so I pulled him up on top of me, and he slid in. My pussy was ready, inviting him in this time. Lubed to the max, all the sensual massage and visual play turned me on even more. He was an animal and loved the crazy party scene (as did I). Moments later, it was hard to bear the heat of the room. Soon, the fun toned down, and I suggested they stay and we go, so they could talk and have some aftercare** discussion without us.

We left with only twenty minutes more to dance, water up, and clean up. Afterward, we continued the evening back at his place. I went down on him while driving home, and when I came back up from his lovely, tasty dick, I said, "I guess this was our first real date!" He smiled and laughed. I said, "What? You opened the door for me ... You were a gentleman." He replied, "That's about all you can tell people when they ask how your first date was!" I smiled and said, "Yup! What else do they need to know besides you were quite the gentleman and opened my door?" ;)

## The Lessons

Don't let your mind insert meaning where there isn't any. You don't know what you don't know, so ... you don't know. Listen to your mind next time and allow yourself to acknowledge why you're thinking that way and nothing more. Don't let it overtake your true self. Making assumptions always puts a damper on the situation. Listen to your internal guides, your gut, and your heart because we are just meaning-making machines ... so drive with your heart, and it will give you a statement. This lesson has to do with the other girl Tristan made out with. I had no idea what they were and only made assumptions based on what I was thinking, which in turn drove me away from him at the beginning. I truly never did ask that night. Was I scared of the answer? Maybe (more like *yes*). Did I want to know? Well, yes and no ... I only did if it was what I wanted to hear at that moment. I was in party mode, not wanting to make any rash decisions, and liking someone that strongly at the start of the game, I had to be careful. I did what most people would do—I hid my emotions and brushed it off (because that's exactly what we should do, insert: slow laugh). I did learn from this, and I hope you do too. This was just a party thing, and he had no intentions towards her.

They were friends, something I found out later in the game. I had to drive him to be more diligent, to be more respectful towards me regarding how he acted around her—because she clearly liked him as well. This caused bad energy between us. Own your worth.

New relationships are awesome and fun—except when you go play without having the conversation about boundaries**— about what we are both ok with. This made it very difficult to even enjoy the experience. Considering we had just started and he wanted to screw around right off the bat didn't rub me the right way. It was both of our faults. It takes two to tango and two to have a conversation. Have it! Be clear and calm; state your worth and values since that's essentially what boundaries are. Sometimes going with the flow can do more harm than good. Speak up because who else will for do it for you? As for that couple, eventually (and I mean years later), we had a discussion with them and around it. They were actually really cool and understood. I haven't had bad communication with anyone yet. I talked to Tristan about that day, and he had no idea. How could he? We were in the "seeing each other" phase and didn't know our body language yet. It was shitty it happened; however, I can say it did, and now I know what to do differently.

If you have a concern about what intentions you have or he/ she/they/all have, just ask. It's that simple. We always make it more complicated than it really is—by putting more behind the conversation. By doing so, we create a wedge and a scapegoat to avoid having the conversation. As Nike said so well, "Just do it!" You will be relieved afterward. Either you're on the same page, or you're not. If you're not, then a least you know and you don't have to waste any more time, or you can create a win-win situation you both agree on. If you are both perfectly on the same page, awesome, brilliant—now go have fun!

# Glossary

*The Corkscrew*: Use your hand up the shaft, going to the top, then gripping at the bottom again and twist—with lube—gently, with slight pressure up, and repeat. For more on blowjobs, a good book is *Heads Up: Increase your sexual confidence, expand your sexual repertoire, and get the real lowdown on oral sex* by Dr. Teesha Morgan and Constance Lynn Hummel.

# 14

# BLINDFOLDED BY NIGHT

⸌He was hypnotic and purely embraced my every sensation. Mystery and wonder were among us, as I had met another as well … Her skin was soft and olive, her movements like a cat. I couldn't get enough of just looking at her, cherishing her. She was gentle and in a flow state—the state of the feminine divine. Her name was Aliza … ⸌

O ne night, after yet another consciousness dinner party where Kava** was poured, the conversations and the people started to dissipate until only five of us were left.

Lying on the couch, Candice spoke up to say it was her birthday. All of us looked around, saying we should do something to celebrate. We all were longing for some fun, I could tell, and I suggested a blindfold and a chocolate avocado mousse tasting; it was left over from the dinner party we had just had.

I stole the suggestion from a Tantra* night we had experienced a couple of weeks prior, where that was done to me. I had been blindfolded, lying on the ground, and chocolate mousse was spread on my lips, neck, arms, boobs, only for it to be licked off by five different people who were petting me and, in my ear, telling me to moan and say how much I liked it. One gently lifted up my shirt and tickled the inside of my pant line with their finger, lowering my pants a bit. Not knowing who it was turned me on so much; I was wet. This was how I knew Candice would love the experience.

When I said, "Blindfold?", everyone said, "Ah YES! Great idea!" and we all scattered to get Candice ready for the pampering. Tristan began first by blindfolding her. He was also the first one to start kissing her, making his way down her neck as she smiled and giggled. As soon as I got back from the fridge, I saw them, and my jealousy instantly started raging. I didn't want this at all. I must have looked angry, like I wanted to kill. I knew this so I hid my expression as I ran downstairs, assessing why this had suddenly come roaring up and why he was the one who'd started it. There had been no talk on our end about what we were both ok with and yet he'd pursued his own pleasure—with Candice's consent, but not with mine.

I made my way into Tristan's bedroom to breathe, to calm myself before I let out the rage monster and started saying or doing something I would later regret (I think I would have maybe slapped him) —something that would just cause grief and would be my inner child's reaction to something that I didn't agree with. So I did what I needed to do and removed myself from the situation to rationalize what I was thinking and to better understand my needs and wants, and why I had so much emotion come up. All the while, my emotions were flooding my better judgment.

Tristan came down to see what was wrong. When I told him, he looked surprised and replied, "Really, you are the jealous one? The one who teaches this?" I said, "I'm not perfect, and yes, I am the one who likes these things. However, I wasn't thinking you were going to kiss her!" Lately, this had been coming up. We talked about it briefly, knowing we were missing out upstairs. Since we had never had this chat before, nor were we really "official," I really didn't feel comfortable with what was happening. I felt like making it "official" would be premature and I would push him away if I did want such a thing. He was being mindful and knew there was something up as well; he could tell without me saying so. He led me into him as he reassured me and took me by the hand upstairs. He was the best at grounding me.

Candice was now lying down on the couch in her bra and black panties. She was a tiny girl in length and in form. She had a tight body, and her petite boobs and butt fit her body very well. James was kissing her as she giggled and squirmed. She was constantly giggling (almost as much as an Elmo stuffy—if you're into furry* fetish). Aliza was putting chocolate mousse on her tummy and licking it off. Once me and Tristan entered the room, we both sat down next to her and Tristan was mindful of my needs the rest of the night, which I felt very bad about. I felt like he was missing out on the action because of me. I couldn't change my feelings, but also knowing that he was telling me the truth—that I had nothing to worry about—made it easier. I trusted his words.

I started kissing and licking, tasting her soft skin as I licked up the fluffy vegan mousse. She would moan, her breath faint, and she would jump every time we surprised her with another spot of saucy seduction. I made my way down to her inner thigh, placing the mousse for Tristan to kiss and lick up. I liked to tell him what to do, instead of him just going ahead and doing it on his own. He obeyed and gently licked up her inner thigh as she swayed and jumped. He smiled at me, and I smiled back, even though how I felt about him scared me. I hid it well (not really).

Candice's clothes slid off so they wouldn't get dirty with the mousse (*cough, cough*—yeah, that was sooo the reason why). Aliza got undressed and joined in, then James; eventually, we had a sexy underwear party (cue Quagmire saying "giggity giggity"). Candice was naked now, and the blindfold came off when Aliza went down on her. James was kissing her, and Tristan and I were still slathering mousse on her naked body. We all stopped to talk about our boundaries**, and Aliza said, "Well, I have none." Tristan said, "I have none either," with a smile. Confused, I looked at him, as what he'd said had an impact on my boundaries. Staring at Tristan, I said, "I have some." James was surprised to hear that. I was grinding my teeth and disregarding my gut feeling. I wondered why others kept pushing or even assumed I had no boundaries when I talk about this stuff and partake. Why is it such a shock?!

We wanted Candice to enjoy her birthday to the fullest, so we pinned her down and tickled her in the process—again, with full consent. Then, Candice whipped around and proceeded towards Aliza, taking control the way she liked to—by going down on Aliza. Without hesitation, she went straight for her pussy, while Tristan did the same to me. Aliza and I were kissing side by side and looking into each other's eyes while James petted Aliza's body all over, nibbling at her beautiful tits and kissing her neck and lushest parts.

*This has progressed pretty quickly*, I thought, smiling at the beauty in it. Aliza was a goddess, a force of pure, radiant, warrior, badass feminine, and it showed in her persona, in her eyes, and in her body language. The way she moved was hypnotic and I was under her trance. Her moans were subtle and lustful. While I continued to enjoy the tongue-slashing sliding around my clit and pussy lips, we kissed and touched each other till we reached a climax of blissful surrender.

Since it kept trying to convert into a couch bed, the couch decided for us that it was time we all went downstairs. Naked and drifting down the stairs, we made our way after a small water break. James and Candice got started right away. I opened the door to James's room to see Candice riding him and Aliza getting fingered in the process. It was interesting to see with my slight outsider's perspective; Aliza was beautiful and exotic, and she made sounds that made you want to play** with her more.

Tristan and I joined in. He started banging me missionary while fingering Aliza. This again upset me a little, as we had never fully had that conversation, and I wasn't ok. The situation made me uncomfortable, made me think he just wanted to play, and by that, I meant with everyone, including me.

Sexy play time followed me everywhere I went. It was my energy, my vision, and what I liked, but having a guy I was interested in— pursuing a lot—made it difficult. To be honest, I had always been the one single-playing with other couples and not giving a fuck. I could disconnect from my emotions, my thoughts, and just be a body in the moment; even with friends, there would be no emotional connection to it. Then I met Tristan and wanted him in my life as more than just a playmate, more than just a friend. His sexual energy was as high as mine, and it drove my inner animal crazy, so when we played with others, emotions came up.

James asked me why it would be different for me and why did I change. "Don't change," he would say. But, to me, it was my energy. I wanted to give it to Tristan. I had shifted my energy towards him. I wanted to. Once I like someone a lot, that's just what I do. I wanted to give him my attention. And I felt that dispersing my attention wasn't fair to the partner I was with. James had been taken aback by my response, by the terms I was using. James himself was very new to the scene. I had introduced him to it. And he had never seen me when I was fully into another. I no longer send my energy everywhere; to me, that wouldn't be fair to my partner. With a partner, I am more focused. I like having a main partner when we can both have fun together, not separately, because separately, I feel disconnected, and I always want that connection to stay strong.

In James's room, Tristan was kissing me and fingering Aliza, which meant he wasn't paying attention to me anymore, even though we were making out (barely, due to his lack of attention). His kissing went from a passionate flow to a stagnant stop-and-go. Blah. I was turned off by his inability to pay attention to number one (or I should I say I would have liked to be number one). His misdirection and lolling were unsettling. I moved aside and he followed, thank God! He started to pound me from the back, which I loved as he tended to hit the right places with his amazing cock. We both had a clear view of everyone, and I was playing with Aliza, which I actually preferred. He couldn't help himself—seeing what Aliza and I were doing turned him on and seeing it while pounding me was an all-time high. He started to go faster and faster till I couldn't concentrate on Aliza anymore as his movements were throwing off the finger-banging I was giving her. Making my man cum twice was an achievement (*teeheehee*) … He was a freak, and I loved it.

He quickly pulled out to finish on the towel close by; he was a quiet cummer, which was odd. I wondered if he was shy in that department, or had he been told not to? Either way, I wanted to get his inner warrior to take charge and express his deep inner pleasures. I wanted to see his vulnerability through and through.

Looking around, everyone was getting tired and slowing down into a cuddle puddle, so we laid Aliza in bed upstairs and kissed her goodnight, leaving James and Candice to have some more fun alone. After realizing that Tristan likes it downright dirty and sexy, I was depleted and wanted my alone time with him. We went down to his room where we found ourselves completely exhausted, and we were entangled in a deep sleep in each other's arms in no time.

The next morning, I found out that Tristan wanted to fuck Aliza but didn't know where her BF would stand on this. I was like, "Umm no … I am not comfortable with that." I crossed my arms in the process. I was surprised that he thought that would be alright. I was in disbelief and total shock since with any BF, or just fuck friend, I would have the conversation about who we would be fucking. If one wasn't ok with the situation, then one could leave. Or one could be ok with it and the other would know what was up and so on and so forth. But the trouble here was that there had been no conversation or even any consideration towards my feelings at all, which in turn made me wonder yet again why this person was doing this. It almost felt as if I was the one who had been blindfolded and not seeing the flags in front of me …

Everyone looked surprised at how my boundaries had shifted.

Or rather were revived. They looked at me as if I should be open to anything and everyone ravishing me since they had no idea what I wanted in a relationship beyond just pure sex. What I said to James was how I truly feel. I wish there had at least been a conversation about the fact that he was fucking me and wanted to fuck others, or seeing me and seeing others. I adored him, and I had thought that, because of his age, he would have known to have these conversations. I gathered my things and left to go home to rest, rest, and rest some more. That night had stirred up some sexy questions. Nonetheless, it was one hell of a night to remember …

## The Lessons

When your man decides to go ahead and start kissing another *again*, I think it's time to have that chat about what you're comfortable with and what you're not comfortable with or what is ok and not ok in terms of your boundaries. As the night progressed, it still wasn't clear what our boundaries were even after Tristan said I was just being jealous. But really, was I? My boundaries were being pushed, my voice wasn't being heard, and we had never had that conversation about what we were ok with. I did realize that we hadn't had that conversation yet because I didn't want to scare or push him away—how silly of me. Would you want to be with someone who would be scared of what you had to say? If you respect yourself, the answer is no. But yes, I did do this to an extent and so I learned from it. I'll be the first to say I'm not perfect; no one is. Even when you teach this stuff, you cannot see what you don't know, and you cannot know what you *don't know*. That being said, sometimes an outsider can see what is going on more easily than you yourself can, which is why check-ins and chats are so important.

Disconnection from one's body isn't right—at all. I used to do this all the time in order to please others or to simply stop caring so I could just enjoy a situation without considering the impact on others' feelings. Trust me, it's not the right thing to do. People are not just skin and bones; they have hearts and souls. Treat them as such, as you want to be treated as well. When you disconnect from your body, you can also have a harder time reconnecting to yourself again and may have to re-learn how to do so. You will have to reconnect with your body and internalize your sensations in order to feel yourself once again. Meditate to zone in on your subconsciousness and conscious awareness, and to be present for your breath, your heart, and your inner cells moving through your body. Just by being in your body, you can re-sensitize yourself and reconnect. It takes time and patience, but it's worth it. There are also sexual practices for healing as well: OM* or orgasmic meditation, sexual healing massages*, tantric healing practices and more.

Furthermore, I think I discovered more about myself in this process. For example, I'd always thought of myself as bisexual* when, in fact, I am bi-situational*. I was always bi-curious*; I was heterosexual but interested in sexual experiences with the same sex. However, not all women turn me on or get a *wow* outta me. The situation is important as well—how things can flow. Some women I would love to ravish, and others I really just like to look at and admire. Brains and personality are big factors for me. If you're ugly on the inside, you're ugly to me.

Lastly, your inner guide—once again, trust it. I was just starting to re-recognize my true intuition and slowly accept how strong and powerful it is. When your guy says he has no boundaries after you just talked to him about yours, you have a red flag on your hands. Tristan still didn't recognize what I felt comfortable with, nor did he hear me. Yet again, he wasn't truly mine.

Make peace with your adventures and see them as opportunities to grow when things arise; rather than doubting and ruminating, learn from the situation and move on. You'll be doing yourself a favor.

# Glossary

*Bi-curious:* A heterosexual person who is interested in sexual experiences with a person of the same gender. This could be in a fantasy context, play context, or another context.

*Bi-situational:* A heterosexual person who is interested in sexual experiences with another person of the same sex, depending on the circumstances and situation, a.k.a. "mostly straight."

*Bisexual:* Those who identify as bisexual feel a sexual and/or romantic attraction to people of a different gender or of the same gender. This term gets tossed around a lot, even for those who are only bi-curious. A.K.A. "Bi."

*Furry Fetish:* Getting turned on by dressing up in an animal costume, still with human capabilities.

*OM:* Orgasmic meditation is a practice of nest building, one-way touch or fully receiving every sensation. The touch is a mindful pleasure in which the giver uses a certain technique with the receiver, like playing a violin. OM usually lasts around 15 minutes, and it involves slow, consistent, but small—barely touching!—strokes of the clitoris. I bet you haven't heard about that one! And yes, it can he healing and a full-blown release!

*Sexual Massage:* Involves one-way touch as the masseuse only touches you. This touch is whole-body and does not exclude any part of the body unless discussed ahead of time. Sexual massage is used to help overcome sexual trauma through safe, consensual touch. It is slow, soft, and sensual but includes some pressure. A full-body orgasm or just an orgasm can happen. Sounds are encouraged to express pleasure.

*Tantra:* In Sanskrit, the word "tantra" means "woven together," and the aim is to achieve mindfulness and deep connection for its participants through breathwork, extended eye contact, embraces, massages, and slow, present intercourse. Tantra can occur with or without sex. Involves energy work.

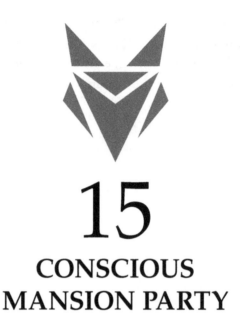

# 15

## CONSCIOUS
## MANSION PARTY

‑A house dedicated to the luscious sounds, movements,
medicines, and ongoing ceremonial pleasures.‑

We had been at a dinner party, so when we arrived, we were dressed as such, and I stood out like a sore thumb. My dress was black and tight—made by Guess—and it turned heads. As I made my way in, saying hi to everyone I knew, I kept getting compliments on my looks.

In the painting room—a.k.a. the dining table—to our immediately left when we walked in, a spread was laid out on the floor, where five others were bringing their visions to life with brushes. In the kitchen, chocolate edibles were placed in order, each with a tag detailing the types of effects and their potency. We danced past the kitchen island into the living room, where the drum circle resided. The mansion had hidden rooms, so we went to explore them and the cuddle fests taking place within them.

It all started in Sage's room, a wonderland where massages and cuddling were on full display. His room was a paradise, a large sanctuary overlooking the backyard. The space, all by itself, was worth remembering for the sunrise the next day. Bamboo lined a wooden pathway over a seemingly endless pond; it was as if you had entered into a different world altogether. Mist and butterflies were the only thing missing from such a perfect scene, but hummingbirds fluttered past the window.

I was lying on the floor cross-legged, looking at the ceiling with a girlfriend of mine, giving her free coaching advice on how to ease her mind and keep her overthinking at bay. She was giggly and intense, so I told her to relax into me. Holding on to emotions that made no sense in the moment, she just wasn't present at all. I could feel the electric sparks of her energy misfiring in all directions, giving meaning where there shouldn't be any. She wanted help embracing her sexual essence—her radiance, her inner sex goddess. She had it in her, but it was blocked by fear, needy desire, and an attachment style** that generated fear and anxiousness. I felt for her as I lay there with her. I got up so I could sit beside her and pet her. Then I added another to just pet her, and I encouraged her to close her eyes so she could embrace the experience, all the while making sure she felt safe and secure. I also kept checking in to see that she was still present for the energy and connection in front of her.

She started to let go and feel again. I felt her body sway more into her femininity and start to release, but so far only in moments. She was too in her head, or in her masculine energy, to receive, let go, and just flow. We continued with more petting, and then cuddling, until I asked to take my leave of the situation. She acknowledged my request and allowed another to proceed. I trusted that individual, but I gave him guidance and set the rules for her healing process to keep moving forward.

I had seen Tristan petting and murmuring to Britney, so I

staggered over to the bed to join in the six-person cuddle fest—to just be and hold space. I relaxed into Tristan's arms, feeling at ease, feeling as if I could be there forever, always in his embrace. I smiled as it was heavenly. Beside us, Britney was mumbling about some documents she needed, her eyes glazed in half-sleep. We went along with it and answered her, babbling back and forth, telling her a man had gotten the documents. She replied, "Ok, we need to go," and we all looked at each other and said, "Where?" She mumbled something else and rolled over. Everyone else looked confused and soon departed the conversation, checking in with Britney before moving on.

I decided to make my way downstairs to the basement where a DJ was jamming and a hula girl was ripping up the floor. I started dancing away with James. Tristan left briefly to bring Aliza to the party while I caught up on some much-needed dancing. While trying to go low in my tight black dress, I wished I'd had a flowy dress on or even pants at this point. I said "Fuck it" to people, no longer caring how high my skirt would go.

An hour later, Tristan made it back, and I pulled him into a cubby hole hidden away for some desired sexy time. The cubby was off to the back of the dance floor, away from lights and lurking eyes. When I plopped myself inside, he said, "What … Where is this leading to?" I smiled, and he climbed in, taking me for all I was worth and loving it. The pumping bass from the music and the drum circle beating down from above made for an epic beat-bass momentum in such close proximity to our sexual embrace.

Our moments are always *moments*, never dull as we always make things interesting. Our heavy breathing and my screaming moans of pleasure went unheard. When we looked around, no one was on the dance floor; we were the only two fully indulging ourselves in the music. I could feel his energy shifting, entwining with mine. He was a powerful force, and I embraced it with every sense. Back to reality after our private sensual dance, he pulled away and swept off to fetch Aliza, but I wanted to stay downstairs dancing, so I kissed him goodbye. It wasn't long before the room started to fill again.

Making my way back upstairs for some conversation, I made sure to say hi to people I had missed at first. I met some new faces and encountered some old when I joined a cuddle puddle on a mattress next to the fireplace. (With the type of crowd at these play parties, it is common for there to be blankets and mattresses on the floor everywhere.) The guy next to me, Tony, said there was something unique about me. Smiling, I said, "Yes, and soon there will be eight … eight to ten." He raised his brow and laughed after asking if that was code for something. I replied, "You will soon see," and smiled mischievously. I got up and walked away, my vision of what was to come playing in my head.

Around the corner, I found Aliza and attacked her with hugs and kisses; she embraced my gestures of love towards her. She is a beautiful goddess, through and through. Her heart is gold, and her sharp mind doesn't get disturbed by society's ways. Smiling after my welcoming embrace, I rushed her to Sage's room for more.

I plopped her on the bed, where she lay in the middle of all of us, for a relaxing petting zoo session. I had suggested—with her consent—that we pet her. She smiled briskly, and I explained that everyone was to be mindful and that this was a "petting only" session. My mind was becoming dreamy as I looked around the bed and counted eight. I smiled. Tony, in disbelief, started laughing and said, "No way … how … whaa …" Still smiling, I said, "See? I told you." I winked and stuck out my tongue, all cutesy.

As the petting got underway, Tony grabbed Aliza's boobs. She looked shocked. I told him that was not ok and asked Aliza if she was ok. She replied, "Yes … but I wasn't ok with that." I turned to Tony to explain that consent was a major factor and that he must ask to touch. I made him understand that this act was not ok. Tony apologized quickly. After that, Aliza snuck off after everyone started progressing on to each other rather than just on her. James and Candice were cuddling, and others expressed intent towards each other. Tristan and I again made an exit to our hideaway; we only had to glance at each other to know.

Grinning, we made our way down (basically running there) and hopped into our hiding spot. Only two people were dancing on the dance floor, but it didn't matter. We didn't care if others saw us, nor did we care if others watched. We liked putting on a show. The music still acted as a cover to any noise we made in the process.

Passionately kissing, I unbuckled and unzipped his pants before reaching down and gently pulling out his cock to hit my throbbing wet pussy. He wanted to penetrate me—all of me. He had been lusting after me just as much as I was after him. He lifted up my dress and pushed my panties aside. I reached down to grab the padded floor, only to find condoms. "How convenient!" I said, smiling like a magician. I handed them over to Tristan. He looked as if I had just pulled them from my bra. Chuckling, he ripped one open and put it on right away, so he could stick it to me like no other. I was soaked for him. He had that effect on me. He was on top, my legs wrapped around him, interlocking us. I grabbed his ass to go in deeper, and I squirmed with pleasure. A couple sneaked a peek and said, "Oh, sorry, guys … uhh …" Tristan replied, "No worries, we don't mind at all," and smiled at me. I smiled back. (It's true; we loved it and loved seeing people get pleasure from watching us). The lights flowed over us, and each song guided our sexual polarity**. Intermeshed with each other, we pounded our way through song after song until we got parched and needed to take a break. But we agreed to come back down soon and winked at each other.

Tristan and I removed ourselves for a fourth time to attend to our required sensations downstairs. Afterward, exhausted and full, we went back to Sage's room and joined the cuddle fest that had been ongoing as if we'd never left. After throwing myself on the bed, I saw Dariel from across the bed and wrapped my arms around him in a full body hug/cuddle. He was a dear friend and a major hippie, all about peace and against negativity. True to his name, Dariel was a shining light; he always embraced everyone with warmth and a smile.

Sitting up, Tony asked if anyone wanted to try some love drug—sassafras* he called it. I've only seen this around a few times; usually it is cut with other things, so it can't really be trusted. I asked how strong it was, and Tony replied, "It's strong but not overly." I looked at its brown, crystal-like form and said I would take a small amount since I am very sensitive to drugs. After dabbing a bit on my finger, I sucked it down. There was no burning or aftertaste or other sensation. It was pure and pleasant, and it hit us like a warm, blissful hug that eases your whole body into an erotic ecstasy.

Half-an-hour later, me and Tristan went downstairs for a fifth time, seeking our private haven, openly touching each other along the way, leaving a sexual energetic charge behind us. Giggling, we shuffled our way down, feeling the effects of the crystals throughout our bodies; it amplified the tantric flow in our touches and in our movements. On our way down, we noticed the music was absent. After pushing over twenty buttons and fiddling with knobs, the drag-and-drop method was the winner. Joking about "an AME and an electrical engineer entering a DJ booth," we laughed out loud at the simple joy that was our silliness.

We did a humble dance before we seductively started moving towards the cubby. Tristan lifted me up and in, and he followed, yet again ravaging me, but in a slower, sensual way. We became more emotionally connected with every kiss we shared, every touch and graze of fingers lingering their way down and around. I moved with every kiss and touch, even the slightest. My heart pounded; my eyes desired more. I pressed him to continue, making it hard to even think about the world outside our intense bubble. Time wasn't there, nor was our ego. No thoughts or external surroundings. We were just present in our embrace.

Holding each other before calmly slithering our way out, we were again interrupted by the DJ. He hadn't known how the music had come on until he saw us. Laughing, he said, "I should have guessed." We smiled at each other. I adjusted my dress, and we made our way back upstairs to see people moving towards the bed to massage others. Three people were about to be massaging one who was getting all the attention (Heaven, right?).

The bed was still full-ish. Knowing I was about to run off, James pounced on me and asked, "Ok, where are you two going? I tried finding a place for me and Candice but can't seem to find one." Smiling, I took his hand and showed him. He smiled back and hugged me. He and Candice went to the same spot that Tristan and I had used for our sexual trips in the past few hours. Now we would be joining the massage people after securing consent. Tristan took Britney in his arms, and she wrapped her body around him. They moved towards the stairs. Confused, I looked at him; his leaving with her troubled me. For one, he was embracing someone else and not telling me what was going on. My mind was bound to wander, especially with her. After a while, he returned, once again with her in his arms. She was smiling, nestled in his embrace. Naturally, I was suspicious, so I asked where he had gone. He replied, "Took her to the bathroom." I wondered why she didn't just go alone. *Why couldn't she ask a female? Why did she ask him and not Brandon (the one she had come with)?* He then said, "She couldn't walk." I couldn't believe her—that she would get so fucked up, she would need help. This was an actual occurrence. I was not impressed, but a purer form was guiding me to seek bliss and non-conflict.

After they got back, I went to the bathroom to cool off, even though I felt barely able to move. I said I was ok, so Tristan left it at that. He was on the bed with Britney and the others. I could barely get up the stairs. When I made my way back, I saw Britney and Tristan on the bed, and I tried to sit next to them, but there was no room in between. (Yeah, I know—I would be wedging them away from each other.) I was uncomfortable with how close they were. With my hands, I willed Britney's half-asleep body to move. She was unaware of my full presence because she was asleep, leaving herself open. Her body was an empty vessel and it showed. She moved where I made her, and Tristan looked at me in amazement. I looked at him in acknowledgement. (I already knew I was a healer, but I did not want to tell anyone as I had work to do myself.)

After she woke up and left, Tristan and I got closer, fully into each other. Smiling, we slowly pulled off our clothes, undeterred by where we were—only enjoying our bodies, our fullness, along with our emptiness (depending on how you view it). We flowed with the music that quietly played on in the background. Tony entered while Tristan and I were playing. We looked at each other with dreamy eyes and knew it was *on*. Two became three: Tristan doing me from behind while I went down on Tony; Tony going down on me as I went down on Tristan; Tristan doing me from behind against the wall while Tony watched and played with himself. The sounds I made told him I loved it. I grabbed Tristan's ass for more, making it obvious that I liked it deep, pounding into me. Grasping for more, I breathed in. We were entangled in each other's sexuality. I loved it when Tristan grabbed my hair every so often to pull me in. Tony smiled and asked if he could join in more, but I said "umm" and told Tristan I only wanted him right now. Tristan told Tony we were going to just rest and cuddle together alone for a bit (to reconnect).

That's what we did. On the floor, I rode on top of him, then kneeled for a moment to kiss gently but passionately in our own world, our internal dream haze. He plopped me down on the floor with him, and I cradled my legs around him, smiling and relaxing. We were ourselves once more. Before we could fully enjoy it, Britney opened the door and inserted herself in the middle of the two of us. She tried hugging and holding Tristan, leaving me on the outskirts. *Not cool!!* I thought big time. I wasn't able to muster up a conversation or tell her to back off as we were both naked head to toe. I was not at all impressed with her actions. And it bothered me that Tristan did not say anything. I thought, *Really?* I looked at Tristan, trying to get him to get her off, but he just looked at me, smiling. I rolled my eyes. I knew Britney was in love with Tristan, and Tristan was acting blindsided, but I didn't know how to talk about it. When I realized he had to make a choice, I felt disrespected and unheard. In this moment, I also felt unseen, so I left.

While I cooled off in the bathroom, he went to check up on me and give me a hug, which progressed to us going downstairs to chat and be together once more. We had sex more than eight times up and down those stairs, and our alone time had always been cut short by someone. I made my way upstairs to curl up next to the fireplace. The sun was shining in my face, so sleep was not on the agenda. I passed some kids fixing their cereal, me with only a t-shirt on. I pulled it down to cover my privates while I got my clothes together. I realized we were the last ones there. When I opened the door, the fresh air was a pleasure and I flushed.

Tristan hugged me goodbye. He was taking Britney home. I went to find the rest of my things before journeying home myself. When I got home, I embraced my bed, flopping down with a smile. Half an hour later, Tristan called. "You home?" he asked. "Yes," I said. He replied, "I'll call you back in 15 minutes." I looked at the time after we hung up. Half an hour went by before the doorbell rang. I smiled as I knew who it would be. I opened the door to a warrior, a man, a lover holding a bouquet of flowers. He had just come back from a sweat lodge ceremony. He apologized for not having the time to cuddle with me. I almost teared up—in my PJs, my hair ragged, smiling. Tristan then gave me an hour to get ready to spend the day with him. I couldn't resist, and I did not want to. He wanted to spend time with me, and treasure our moments as well ...

## The Night Full of Lessons

Unless you coach people for a living, or for fun like I do, please don't take it upon yourself to help people open up. A lot can come up for certain individuals, especially dealing with sexuality. For example, did you know that Marilyn Monroe went through a traumatic event?

One that affected her sexuality? She eventually realized that if she rubbed her clit with Saran Wrap on a man's tailbone, she would feel safer and be able to cum. From there, she progressed to skin-on-skin, rubbing only her clit, until she felt more comfortable—and with a person she felt comfortable helping her.

Pain can come up, along with anxiety, or a strong case of the giggles … You get my point. Stuff comes up, and being naked (not that that's where you're going to end up right off the bat) is being pretty fucking vulnerable, if you ask me.

When creating a "petting zoo," make sure you establish solid boundaries** and/or ask what each individual's boundaries are since some might not speak up for themselves. In Aliza's case, there had been no chat about it beforehand; it had only been communicated that we were only allowed to pet, that's all. After that, we began, and then someone grabbed in an area that had not been ok'd. At that point, boundaries were laid out, but it is always a good idea to have the discussion beforehand to try to minimalize these types of incidences. Neither party knew the set rules or didn't speak up. When I saw that, I spoke up for them. Check in or check the fuck out.

When a woman gets the guy you're seeing to help her in the bathroom, and your man doesn't tell you until afterward, that's a red flag, and this one was on Britney. She knew she can ask another woman to go with her, or she could have asked the guy she'd come with, but no—she asked the guy I was seeing. And when they came back, she was in his arms, hanging on him and nuzzling. No, I didn't do anything at the time because I didn't know what the situation was, and I had to process why she was so keen on Tristan all the time. All the clues added up—she was totally into him, and later on, she was trying to get in between Tristan and me while we were cuddling naked. (Not cool, Britney, not cool.) She didn't ask; she just jumped in when we were trying to have a moment for ourselves. I left in discomfort and feeling disrespected by Britney. I was still trying to find my voice at the time myself.

That said, having a discussion with her would have only led to disaster as I had tried before. So, Tristan took it upon himself to have a conversation with her to make sure she knew that he and I were together. Thanks, love!

Sex! Yes, please! More please … What a wonderful thing! Sex relieves stress and depression, and it lowers cortisol levels, boosts the immune system, and releases oxytocin. It even burns calories, among other things! So, why not have sex? Well, only have it when consent is expressed, and when protection is available (unless you're with a partner you trust and have been with for a while). Even in play mode, make sure to have contraception close by, making it easy to grab when you're in the moment. I am a firm believer in sex and play**, the latter a term I use that means everything up to oral (but not penis in vagina). Have fun, and be safe and consensual!

Playing in three's: My guy is a freak in the sack, and I love it! We are both always playing and exploring, but when it comes to playing with others, be careful as you can catch stuff, even through oral sex. The most common sexually transmitted disease is chlamydia*, which is super easy to treat and get rid of (Go to your doctor for a test or prescription medication). When you're into the lifestyle, it is common to get tested every month or so, depending how much you play, swing, or have sex.

Once the party was over, my mind wouldn't stop thinking about how Britney kept trying to get Tristan's attention all night by doing little things (yes, that pissed me off). Even though she said she respects me, if she truly did, she wouldn't have done the things I talked about above. She also said that Tristan had only bought me flowers to balance my energy out because he felt bad about driving her home and leaving me. She told me not to read too much into it, as "it was only a nice gesture." I looked at her in disbelief because I knew the true reason. She even tried to tell me that he didn't want to be in a relationship and that's why she didn't pursue him. I knew then where she was coming from, and I knew in my gut that the words Tristan had spoken were genuine and kind. There was no hidden meaning, nothing about "balancing my energy." He had shown up. Again, remember to listen to yourself because that's where the truth lies.

# Glossary

*Chlamydia:* A sexually transmitted disease that is more common than some would think. There may be no symptoms, or there may be discharge and/or a burning sensation while peeing and/or swelling. Best to ask your doctor and get checked. And use protection!

*Sassafras:* A pure form of drug extracted from a rare plant. The sensation resembles that of being on molly. Molly is MDMA, which is a chemical of sensory input that dumps feel-good receptors—serotonin, dopamine, and norepinephrine.

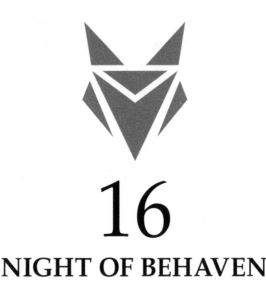

# 16

# NIGHT OF BEHAVEN

~We were all going to BEhaven at Expressions for the first time. Seven of us piled into the event and danced to three different room beats. The fourth room was the dungeon and playroom. Attire was mandatory for this room, so I dressed Tristan up in a collar, with two tie-downs attached for me to pull on (highly recommend, by the way!) like reins. Here we go … fetish, the LBGTQ community, sin, play, and the burner crowd all in one party!~

We knew we were gonna get frisked upon entry, so boob and pussy storage it was! Tiffany had asked me to stuff a bottle of something up my pussy in order to get it in; she was on her period so she couldn't. I agreed, and we all got searched, frisked, and whatnot. Good thing we had stashed everything before trying to get inside. We just had top-ups in our bras. Thinking we were so sly, I smirked.

Once inside, Tiffany and I went into the bathroom. I tried to dig out the bottle I'd hidden, but I couldn't grab it. The situation was intense. I started to panic. Tiffany got down, her hands deep inside me. She thought she would have to call the ambulance. I told her, "No, go deeper. I can handle it. Have you seen Tristan?" Laughing and anxious, she told me to brace myself, and oh-my-god, she went elbow-deep into my pussy as if I were giving birth. She asked if I was ok. I said, "Yeah, just give me a second." We were so close to calling someone to come get the thing outta me, but we finally got it, thank God! Laughing, I splashed water on my face, and Tiffany and I looked at each other in a did-that-just-happen kinda way before we said, "Let's go!"

We were greeted by jungle beats, EDM, and techno/dub/trap. Dress attire was barely there, not enough for me to dance my true range of motion, get into the flow of the music, or to work up to any sexual escapades. We moved into the bigger room where there was a cirque performer, flashing lights, and a full swing of people enjoying the beats. I beelined to the black birdcages at the back of the dance floor. Tiffany and I both held the reins to Tristan's collar, and we led him into the cage for dancing and fondling. Every so often, we would pull him in to kiss, dance, or fondle. His eyes gleamed at the exciting scenery and open play**. Tiffany and I danced exotically around him, touching and making out with each other, and popping our asses into each other's hands. We couldn't help but touch each other; we loved it. Tristan grinned with amusement when Tiffany and I stuck our asses out to be flogged** by a random spectator who made perfect figure-eights on our asses. Once again, I was in heaven (Have I mentioned that I loved being flogged?) as the long leather straps hit our cheeks in a fast-grazing way. Tristan couldn't help but miss me. He loved seeing me pleasured. Getting flogged heightened my endorphins, the thudding wisp of the leather and the dominant nature of the one behind the flogger.

The girl said thank you by kissing our asses (yes, she asked beforehand), and we moved onward, finding the play den and putting on one hell of a show for all to see! First, we made our way over to the big play pad, as big as two king size beds, saying hi to everyone we recognized mid-play. We hustled over to the far side so I could watch Tiffany and get pounded from behind while I made out and fondled her from the other side of the ledge. It was hot as hell, and yes, we got complimented by others ("Wow, she really likes it rough" or "She loves getting pounded, doesn't she?"). Tristan would smile, and my muffled moans and pleased expression said it all. I couldn't help it; I loved him, loved his cock, his eagerness, his warrior essence, and our sexual polarity**. We always amazed each other, it seemed, and loved our voyeur personas.

I reached around to grab his ass and push him further into me. I wanted him, all of him, and I wanted it now. He then went full force, driving into me like no other. I was on cloud nine and couldn't resist cumming twice from such hard, pleasurable action. He spun me around and plopped me gently on the floor, and I licked and sucked, tickling his balls every so often while playing with his huge erect dick and looking up at him in awe. He smiled and then pushed me down. I loved it when he took charge because I could be in my feminine zone, more open and free for him to just take me.

He kissed me and I grabbed the reins to pull him in more. I was getting used to them (I will definitely use these again … Good idea, Z! *hehe*). I could feel his passion with every kiss, every touch, and I knew he was with me, connected; our surroundings didn't matter. He moved down and started kissing my inner thigh as I added slack to the reins. He knew I loved it since my body was moving in for more. Then he looked up at me, his ass in the air, and I saw some guys starting to grab his ass without consent. I kicked them off and said *no, no* with a simple tsk-tsk finger and a smirk. They tried again, and I kicked them off again, this time with a better glare that said, "Back off, bitches" (*hehehe*, yes, that's a look). Dang, they were pushy! I knew my man has a great ass but come on!

Once he made me cum for the third time, he wanted me even more. He grabbed a condom, bent me over, and fucked me good.

Again, I grabbed him for more. I could feel his pulsating dick growing harder at the peak of ecstasy. He was about to blow so I pulled in harder, scratching his back and bringing him in closer. He clenched, flopped over, and held me. I loved it when he did this—his skin, his touch, his scent, and his cumming sensations.

By then, we were parched and the only ones left on the pad. We tapped Myra and James into the play pen. Taking a break on the couch, I was approached for a dance by Dane (He was a mate I made out and danced with earlier this year, which led to a foot massage to die for … Later, I met his GF at a party he had invited me too, and it was a little awkward). I looked over at my man to see if it would be ok. He said, "Go ahead," in an I-don't-care kind of way. I looked at him again to find some comfort in the situation, but none could be found.

Dane and I were off. He was drunk and wearing his fur-and-leather Viking outfit, the one I'd met him in. I was wearing my black mesh tutu, which he loved. We danced on stage for a few songs. He twirled me around and kept peck-kissing me. I could smell his booze-ridden breath, and I kept myself turning, half-laughing at his drunken behavior and half-looking around for Tristan. Hula performers were on stage with us to the left, and there was another performer on her own stage, in a full, fairy-themed aerial get-up. I decided to hug Dane off, say goodbye, and make my way back to Tristan, but I couldn't find him anywhere.

I looked around every room for him—every bathroom, every corner. Thirty minutes went by, and he was nowhere to be found. I was concerned, and my brain was telling me nasty stories about him having gone off with someone else. I asked around, and others said that he had left or that he had gone into the playroom. I wanted to make sure he didn't leave, so I finally made my way to the car.

I found him with Tessa, his friend from out of town. As I approached the car, they were coming around from the back of it, her pulling up her pants and him readjusting and buckling his belt. Not wanting to know anything, my mind going off in all directions, I dropped my gaze. Did I even want to know? He wouldn't, would he? Then he saw me and smiled as they both came towards me. I was in shock, so I listened after asking him where he had been for the last 35 minutes. I told him I became concerned when I couldn't find him.

He looked at me and said, "You sure you weren't jealous?" I was so sick of that accusation; I felt unheard, and his answering with another question didn't justify why he was coming back out from the car. "I didn't know where you were and that scared me, considering you left and weren't in the club," I said, concerned and being cautious as well. He hugged me and kissed me. Maybe I overreacted, but at the same time, usually when you go somewhere with someone, you let them know if you are going somewhere else for a bit, out of respect and acknowledgment. But he had not, and I saw what I saw.

Once back inside the club, Tiffany and Gabriel, were rounding up the troops at this point, as it was time to leave.

Twelve people, one apartment, and Kasey Riot music later, Tristan and I were the first ones on the bed in the middle of the living room for play time (*tehehehee*). We smiled at each other, each knowing how the other felt, without question. We started putting on a show for the couple next to us, and then they started showing us their moves. Next, Gabriel jumped in, beaming, and another individual joined the escapade as well.

This after-play-party was in full swing! I was sucking off Gabriel while Tristan pounded me from behind. Gabriel could barely handle himself, saying, "Oh-my-god, girl, you're gonna make me cum in your mouth ... Ohhhkay, slow down for a bit," which made me grin with excitement at the idea that I could make him blow his load in my mouth. Gabriel loved it, and Tristan loved seeing me giving and receiving so much pleasure. It got him hard for more. Tristan then looked over at the other couple; Gabriel was fingering the girl while she sucked off her boyfriend. Suddenly, the boyfriend asked to switch after a brief stare my way.

I wasn't comfortable with it; I am a tad picky who I share with, and we didn't know this couple, nor had we had the cleanliness conversation. Tristan respected that. After a heated session switching and roleplaying with Gabriel and Tristan, the audience on the couches and surrounding areas were gleaming with enjoyment. Tristan and I took a mini-break, grabbing a glass of water from the kitchen and making our way to the bedroom in the back. We soon realized a cuddle session was in play as this was where the other half of the group had been hiding.

Seven were chilling, cuddling, and slowly starting to play. Tristan and I moved into it, and as soon as we hit the bed, Tristan went down on me, making me grin and moan, not wanting him to stop. Then Tiffany interrupted so she could go down on me. She wanted to surprise me with more action and play down there while Tristan kissed me and watched, getting hard in the process. Then I got asked to play by another. After making sure his girlfriend and Tristan were ok with it, I agreed. He started fingering me while Tristan kissed and held me, and then Tristan grabbed Tessa's boobs in the process. Shocked, I pulled back from him. I was not ok with that. He hadn't asked. He noticed my reaction and said it was nothing, but I was yet again in the position of having to say *he has to ask.*

He kissed me passionately as I moved towards Tiffany, who moved seductively towards me with a question in her eyes. She asked me if it was ok if Tristan pounded her in the ass. She was an ass girl. I thought about it as I switched and crawled on top of Tristan for some bumping and grinding. While he tossed me around, I told Tiffany to give me a second. I was on the edge of the bed with him pounding me more and more, and I couldn't help but dive into it. He fit in me and always made me cum multiple times. I knew Tiffany and trusted her as well. I also knew she wasn't able to play with her v-jay all night due to her moon time, so I told her yes, but I would get to tell Tristan what to do. She said thank you multiple times and hugged me, excitement filling her eyes. I got a kick out of getting to be a part of it, out of knowing I would be the one making it happen—the boss of the situation, the one controlling everything.

I told Tristan he was going to give it to Tiffany in the ass, and he
looked at me and smiled and kissed me. I smiled back, and since he
looked like he was in his head, I asked him what was up. He replied
that he had never done anal before. My smile got wider, and I told
him I was happy I could give him his first time and that it would be
with Tiffany, my girlfriend who I trusted greatly. I told Tiffany out
loud that I trusted her, and Tessa piped up and said, "What does
trust have to do with it?" with a slight attitude in her voice. I smiled
in amazement, and as I was about to answer, someone else answered
it for me beautifully, saying that vulnerability and trust has to be
there in order for a partner to share and be ok with it. Without trust,
you have nothing; no foundation on which to build, no set boundary
control, either. I nodded and added that since I knew Tiffany well,
it helped.

Seven people cheered on Tristan's first time. He also had to rip
the condom off to fuck me a little more to get hard again, which
made my night and made me even wetter for him. Just knowing he
needed me and needed to have sex with me to get hard again—fuck
yeah! Love it! *How sweet*, I thought. We stayed connected by making
eye contact with each other. I loved how he did this for me. It was
something that was missing from our first time together, but it really
helps us keep our connection while playing with other people.

Gabriel asked to pound me, and Tristan and I nodded. He was
quick, but then had to slow down in my pussy. He made a face, and
I could tell he was holding back from cumming in me. He liked my
pussy and made sure I knew it, making sexy comments and making
me tell him I liked it. But I always stayed connected to Tristan. He
pounded Tiffany up the ass till she came. He constantly had to feel
me up and play with me in between to make sure he stayed hard,
which made my body quiver with excitement. Knowing he had to
come back to me for stimulation and connection grounded me,
and I loved it. Our connection grew deeper and deeper from that
point on …

I woke up to a bump and grind that was not Tristan. I said, "nooo," and with Tiffany's support, it stopped. I didn't know where Tristan was, so I started looking around and asking. Tiffany got up and looked too, and she found Tristan and Tessa in the living room. I asked what they were doing. He said they were just talking. In my mind, he should have stayed with me, especially in these types of situations. Had they really been talking or was something happening behind my back? I had to, yet again, not let my assumptions take over. I just wanted to leave at this point. Tristan said he just wanted to chat all night, yet he had yet to do that with me …

## The Lessons

Well, this chapter was a bit of a clusterfuck. A long night of drinking, drugs, and who knows what shenanigans. This Tessa lady and I had just met. Tristan told me we would get along, but little did I know she was over the top, crossing lines like no other. As I mentioned, I had to go looking all over the club for them since they were nowhere to be found for over an hour. Tristan didn't have the common courtesy to tell me either. I finally ventured to the car to find them together in the backseat, doing who knows what. I ran out of there, in the rain, in my tutu, upset and in disbelief over what I had just seen. They both said he had been "helping" her change her shoes (Yeah, I bet!). I was trying to give him the benefit of the doubt.

Needless to say, I never found out the truth, and we had a solid talk about this night. Sometimes you have to be ok with not knowing in order to move ahead. I was not willing to have this experience eat away at me and take up energy better spent on uplifting. I still wonder about that night. Why didn't they tell me where they were going instead of sneaking out for a while? Why did he go with her? Why was he all quiet when he said, "I didn't pull up my pants"? Maybe they were hiding things. She crossed the line again later that night. However, I wasn't going to let their shitty behavior affect mine. I didn't put a stop to the negativity right away, though I wish that had been the case. I practiced unraveling this for a while, asking questions, eventually releasing the unknown to elevate what is important now over what might have been important back then, or what has changed now versus back then. I had to focus on what insight I wanted with me, moving forward into the future.

Now on to the other incident, yay! Grabbing Tessa's boobs when we were clearly seeing each other was disrespectful to me and our relationship. He had just gone for it. I stopped and looked at him in a WTF!? kinda way. Why was there no "Hey, may I?" look or question in my direction? I would not have cared that much. I know they had a past; he had said it wasn't sexual. So why grab her boobs? We had another nice chat about this afterwards. He had thought it was no big deal. Her boobs were fake as hell, she was a friend, and it was not sexual at all; it was just being drunk and on who knows what else. His "hey, let's ask" filter was nowhere to be found.

We continued having a really good conversation around touch, boundaries**, and respecting each other. It really came down to his inexperience with boundaries since his last few relationships were … well … loose cannons and over the top … not much discussion about boundaries since they were both alcoholics and came from trauma … yay (not). That being said, the past does not give them or him a free pass. It just means that where there is more information, more context, and the desire to come forward, there is also the will to learn. Just because you don't or didn't know doesn't mean you won't eventually know. It was a learning curve for sure, and I have to admit, it was hard, but it was worth it. Our relationship really flourished. We've never stopped learning.

As for Tessa, well, she isn't the best at respecting our relationship. It's not her job either. It's Tristan's job. She asked why it wasn't ok for him to grab her boob and what respect had to do with it. On the other hand, Tiffany had asked me what she could do with Tristan, and I know her very well. I didn't know Tessa, and there was no ask. She didn't understand, so I blew her off in conversation and told

Tristan we would talk later. Even though you might think having respect or boundaries should be common knowledge, it's not. Never assume, as this is a taught thing.

As you can tell, I embraced a lot of things in the mood of that night. It was Tristan's first time doing anal sex, and he didn't enjoy it to the point of wanting to do it again. He said, "It was ok," and asked if I had tried anal. "Of course, but I did not find it at all enjoyable," I replied. Needless to say, neither of us are longing for that experience again. I let things slide that night as a one-off and was open to other things—men grabbing Tristan's ass, Tristan having anal with Tiffany, and his leaving the room with Tessa to "chat." A lot happened that night, and I will leave a lot of it in the past. It's great to embrace your mood and yourself as long as you respect yourself and others. When you do that, you stress less, avoid overthinking, and go with the flow.

As a side note, make sure that if you shove something up your pussy, you put a string on it because your pussy might suck it up like mine did. Tiffany had to go fist-diving, scared she would have to call an ambulance. I told her to just get it, and I pushed and pushed, laughing at the innuendo about childbirth. She was elbow-deep, and it took us around 25 minutes, but we got it out. Never again will I make that mistake. At least I know my pussy has a healthy pelvic floor. If you ever need to work on your PC muscles, Kegels* and other exercises could help. Always explore your options, and make sure it's something that will work *for* you and not against you.

# Glossary

*Kegels*: This exercise helps women strengthen their pelvic floor muscles. Kegels can also improve sexual function and treat incontinence. The exercise involves repeatedly contracting and relaxing your pelvic floor muscles; some people use a jade egg (sometimes referred to as a yoni egg) or other device to help with this.

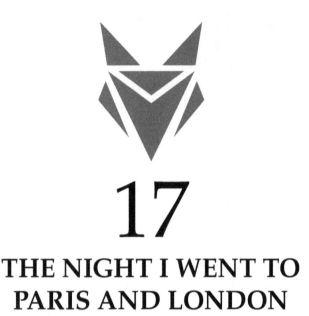

# 17

# THE NIGHT I WENT TO PARIS AND LONDON

~*The Sex Show* is where your sensations and curiosity can explore; where a spanking demo can happen in front of your mom; where a woman called "Grinder Girl" goes on display and expertly eroticizes a big, commercial-grade grinder on metal plates attached to her body for sexual pleasure; where free cam girls run around with their boobs out; and where a really muscular, attractive, 6'1" guy paints with his dick—yes, literally—and sells his paintings; and so much more to ignite your senses before you hit up an after-party to play out your fantasies.~

After a three-day bender of working *The Sex Show*\* and promoting, I was spent; sex toys, lube, intimates; G-spot stimulation seminars, "Sex with Dr. Jess," whip-play workshops—a form of impact play\*, burlesque shows; a "Who has the best ass" competition run by volunteer contestants; and so much more. Attending the event made me realize how vanilla it all was; really, it was more of an introduction to the unknown, the taboo. During my break, I was amazed to see "Grinder Girl" and a very sexy penis painter, who asked for my name. I got his number.

After The Sex Show, Tristan picked me up to go workout and have a nice, relaxing dinner, which turned into having delicious mimosas (and for someone who doesn't really drink much, it was a doozy of an episode after the second one). We splashed back four and snacked on oysters and aged, smoked salmon. We moved on to the next place to munch on waffle fries covered in everything bad—cheese, bacon, ground beef, peppers, tomatoes, and yummy Kelly O'Bryan mayo sauce for dipping, as if our hearts needed more.

On the drive back, I was getting rowdy. I wanted to dance so I said, "Umm … there's an after-party for The Sex Show," to my man, who was sitting next to me. He only smiled in reply. I knew he was down if I was able to handle it. I suggested music—correction: loud music—and a mini dance show while we thought about going.

His friend connected with him, so we invited him along to our potential endeavour. One more drink in and I was ready. The drinks numbed my back, ever-so-done-in by the show as well as my anxiousness about inviting others. I smiled at the prospect of a fun night and got ready, dancing up a storm on my pole in my bedroom to trap deep house music. Tristan pushed me down on the bed for a little play** time before we would have even more play time. I love it when we make sure our personal needs and wants are met by connection together, just us first.

I got him naked first, and we laughed. I always seemed to get him undressed first, even though he tends to try his best to get me undressed and naked all the time. Making my moves, I went down on him. I love his dick, and even more so, how hard he gets for me. His already pulsating boner was ready for action, and I wanted to play. On my way down, I realized I'd gotten straight to it, so I started licking, kissing, and teasing as I danced to the endless list of songs playing in the background.

I truly love him, and every time we are together, another adventure arises, and it is always an adventure, no matter how small or how epic. We play well together, and we work well together, and we are both always passionate in all areas of our lives, something that we strongly support each other in. He is also a true gentleman, be it when he's opening a door for me or holding my hair up while I suck him off.

After spending some time fondling his balls and making it known that I wanted to suck him dry, I slurped him along the way, but he had other plans. He pulled me up by my hair, making me quiver since he knew my tease points, and threw me down on the bed. He remained on the edge of the bed for a better view and better access to my lips, swollen, plump and pinkish red. Sliding his hands along my legs, from my toes to my creamy thighs, he smiled and dove in. He knew I absolutely loved his tongue on my clit. He kissed it gently and blew on it, and every so often, he would lick my luscious lips to tease me, causing me to want more, so I would squirm when I couldn't handle it anymore.

In full swing, I could only see his eyes when I looked down to see him pleasuring me—licking gently and sticking his tongue in and out for momentary penetration. Shaking with excitement and pleasure, I was on the edge, only for him to bring me back down again and then make me moan and grab the sheets once more. Again, he would smile, back off, and reposition himself. He knew I wanted more, but he wanted to take his time before I released my internal fire. He moved his tongue on the length of my clit in full motion, up and down, making me peak. I shook, surrendering all the build-up that I had been edging to let go.

I grabbed his head to bring him up, so I could passionately kiss him as a yummy "thank you." He got on top of me, and I slid his rock-hard cock into me. Feeling him inside of me was another story; his cock felt soft-hard and thick (just the way I like 'em). I grabbed his ass to get him to pound me harder, and he had to stop every so often so as not to blow his load. I smiled at the thought that I could have that effect on him. He grabbed me close, making me stationary, so he could pound me deeper. I couldn't help but let out a sexy sigh and bite my lip to try and not make noise. He flipped me over, putting me on my stomach, because he wanted a better angle. Knowing him, he was about to cum and wanted to prolong it. Stopping and going, I came again, and as I did, he pulled out to release his swimmers all over my tiled floor (Thank God, no carpet).

Getting dressed, I pulled on my tight, stretchy, black-and-white-striped corset, along with a thong, fishnets, and boots. Then I reapplied my makeup for our upcoming nighttime affair. We then picked up Tristan's buddy, which took us into the after-party for The Sex Show. We arrived early, just in time to get one of the beds before it got dirtied up by everyone else's naughty sex-capades, and before the whole place got busy. On our bed, we progressed to fondling and hardcore kissing, taking my thong off for easy access, so Tristan could go down on me once more. Man, oh man, I was in love. He knew how to pleasure me, and hot damn, he's a great kisser.

We moved towards a swing because Tristan wanted to try and make me cum using my G-spot* since we had learned about that at the previous event. He went down on me and fingered me, trying to make me squirt*. Minutes went by, and I was very wet from him going down on me and from seeing him getting more and more excited and intrigued. He then asked the stranger next to us for tips. We tried them out, and Tristan asked the stranger if he could just do everything after making sure it was ok with me. "Game on!" I said. The stranger boasted about how he can make any woman cum and squirt in minutes. He started doing the techniques, and when I realized he was hitting it, it felt weird/awkward/fun without the mind blow.

Tristan was kissing me while the other guy kept going. After about five minutes, he gave up (I guess it is hard to make me squirt). The stranger looked defeated, but Tristan gave him a little gesture and said that I was hard to please, so the guy wouldn't feel so "less than." We thanked him, and he thanked us, saying profusely how beautiful I was. I blushed, acknowledging his compliment. By that time, Tristan wanted in, and we screwed a bit on the swing. Then we moved to the bed below, while Tristan's friend, the squirter guy, and an older, well-dressed Asian gentleman watched. We got even more turned on by creating this display for them. After a heated session, Tristan's legs were cramping from all the thrusting.

We made a break for the dance floor. This place was in the same location as The Dungeon and "Boardshorts or Less." Since it was underground, it was dark and dingy and had that underground vibe. There were beds, swings, condoms, and more. The place got heated fast, since it was a tinier venue, but it had lots of places in which to play around. We only danced for a bit, downing water, until we wanted each other again.

The atmosphere was driving us into seduction. We went to play again, this time next to a couple on the bed. Then another couple joined us while Tristan was pounding me from the back. A blonde wanted in, so I looked at Tristan. He nodded, and then I nodded to her. She went under me, down towards my clit, licking and touching, which drove my senses wild. Below me, she moved up, which made her pussy ripe for the picking, and I gave it a little lick, teasing her, while her playmate was kissing her on the side. He was half-standing, half-kneeling, and watching in awe at the same time. Tristan was getting harder and needed to stop before he blew.

He decided to switch to licking me while I was licking this beautiful, luscious blonde, feeling her movements, moving with her, and listening to what she wanted, how her body was responding. Her breathing got heavier and faster, her breaths shorter. Tristan was licking and penetrating me with his tongue. I was in bliss, in the moment, on the pleasure train of nothingness and everything. After seeing the woman's face release and her army boots kick before relaxing, she thanked me and continued sharing the space while sucking off her boyfriend. Her boyfriend was watching me get pleasured while he was getting it himself. A few more minutes later, I turned around to pay Tristan back for the favor, and we matched the couple next to us. I sucked him off, with a slight twist of my hand as well for extra pleasure. He was deep-throating me, and I handled it well, teary-eyed, drooling, and sucking all at once. My makeup started to look almost "whore-like," my eyeliner smudged by the tears and sweat. Some would find that hot as hell. In fact, I have a friend with this kink**.

Tristan fist-bumped the guy next to us, and I couldn't hold in my laugher at the sight. The blonde and I both burst out in laughter and delighted bliss while freshening up. Afterwards, I went to the bathroom to wipe off my smudged black eyeliner since this was not my kinda kink. I finished freshening up while Tristan waited outside. We decided now would be a great time to rest, refresh, and check in. After dancing and drinking the rest of the night, we decided to leave at 1 am after DJSPANK finished their set.

Tristan, Gabriel, and I agreed to go to Gabriel's for after-play-party fun … 2 am, umm what other ideas had we … high, tipsy, and not wanting the night to end. Mind you, I tasted great … Tristan described my pussy juice as "sweet nectar," and I added in amusement, " …of the gods!" Laughing, he smiled back at me. After arriving, we had a few drinks and put on some more sexy tunes—Kasey Riot's pre-recordings—before touching and feeling and generating the warm fuzzies. Gabriel got the coconut oil out for naked massage time. He always had the best ideas. My back was starting to fuss—it was late after all. Hmm … what could possibly happen with everyone mostly naked and touching each other? Let's find out … I had been honing my inner vixen more and more over time, testing the waters, navigating along the way.

Gabriel was quick—poof!—like magic; he had converted his living room with a mattress and blankets into a space to play and get my body worked on. He invited me down with a gleaming smile. Lying on my stomach, my body instantly wanted touch and movement. Gabriel started on my lower back and moved towards my butt, the asset Tristan was always boasting about, straddling it with his tanned, naked body. Fuck! ... was he in shape, and wow, what a wonderful human being too. As he massaged me, I couldn't help but make noises. Gabriel's dick started tilting upwards along my ass crack. I was feeling it and getting into the groove too. I could feel his shaft pulsing, his dick getting longer, and I was getting turned on by how turned on he was getting. Then Tristan joined in. He started massaging my head and shoulders. He was already pining, thriving with the brilliant seduction of seeing another man touch me. Cuckolding* was his kink—a light form of it. It pleases him to see me get pleased. Since we've been together, his sense of compersion* has become really well developed. His only tick is that no emotional connection trumps the one he shares with me. That is a solid boundary** on his end. Sometimes, just talking about me having sex with another guy is all he really needs to get into the mood.

Tristan was hard, enjoying Gabriel's comments about my "lovely, plump ass" and "velvety skin," while he slid his hands from my ass to my shoulders and back, along my midsection and on down. Tristan was trying to get in on it. He needed recruiting and my necessary hands of encouragement. Gabriel kept going, his dick gliding up and down my ass crack, ever so gently. He was making a face that told me he was practicing orgasmic control*. I wasn't complaining—I was getting pampered like a goddess, slathered in oil, four hands on me and tongue too. They gave me water after the play session, making sure I was taken care of.

It was 3:48 am when Tristan's friend Jay decided to come over. He had stayed at the last party till the end, and now he was, for sure, in for a show. Soon things escalated. I kept rubbing my ass up and down and started giving Tristan a hand job. Gabriel asked if he could use his fingers to penetrate me, and feeling sassy, I said, "You can use more than just fingers." We had played before, and Tristan had given me the go-ahead wayyy in advance for this. He said, "You can do whatever you want with Gabriel, ya know. You have my full consent." If that wasn't an ask and a push, I don't know what is. I was in overdrive. The sensual play* was making me desire more.

Gabriel started with his fingers, lightly massaging me, gliding over me, all juiced with coconut oil for lubrication. From underneath, he rubbed my clit in circular motions, light and luscious, and my sex was turned on, my clit erect. His fingers swirled on top of my clitoral hood and down again, creating pressure from the top with the weight of his body. He lowered himself down to my ear and whispered, "You like that?" I moaned, "Ooh, yeah," my breath heavy.

Gabriel continued rubbing my clit, and Tristan motioned me over towards his cock. I teased him with a gentle lick and twist of my tongue. Jay was sitting on the couch, and Tristan asked him if he was good before asking him to join. I backed up slyly, giving Tristan a cue that I was not down for that since we hadn't discussed it. I wasn't ready or really wanting that, either. Tristan looked at me and shut it down right away. Yes, I have "looks," and killer ones I might add. Jay was loving the show. He liked to watch and was getting turned on just seeing it all in action. This allowed me to be my free, exhibitionist** self, who loved putting on a show.

Tristan and Gabriel flipped me gently onto my back. I was fully exposed now, longing for their dicks. I started to suck on Tristan's thick cock as if it were the first time I had tasted it. I glided my tongue along his shaft. His veins pulsated with pleasure. Gabriel got the go-ahead and tip-teased my sex, rubbing me with his head, sliding it in slightly, saying "Oops" and "Oh no," playfully tease me into wanting more. My hips started to talk more about their longing and desire. Through the sway and rising, I wanted more than a tease, I wanted to be devoured. He kept teasing, and I got wetter and wetter. Testing the waters, he slipped two fingers inside me, pulled out, and slipped them in again. "You're soaking, umm ..." Gabriel bit his lower lip and sucked my juices off his fingers with a slight pop sound. He told Tristan how sweet I tasted, and Tristan smiled, getting more and more excited to see me getting pleasured.

Gabriel slid right in, and I stopped sucking to enjoy taking his cock. I moaned for more. "You want it?" Gabriel would say, and I loved how expressive he was with his teasing. I nodded, and he pounded into me once, stopping to see my sex squirm. I was high, high on life, high on endorphins, and a second wind came on. Gabriel loved to start and stop. He loved the power play of orgasmic control. Tristan watched, his kink growing a little more, playing and loving it. Gabriel went again and again. We must have been at it for ten minutes, me sucking and Gabriel pounding my lustful, thirsty pussy.

Then Gabriel piped up and slowed down. We were all sweaty and all breathing heavy. "Let's switch," he said, and Tristan replied, "Hey, that's my favorite phrase." He smiled gleefully. While Gabriel pulled out and took his condom off, I spun around, but Tristan stopped me with a dominating hold on my throat. He knew how much I loved his masculine side, me in orgasmic bliss and him taking me. Kissing me passionately, he was holding my throat just the way I liked it. I love breath play* and the thrill of the hold. He gripped both sides of my throat with just the right pressure, not in the center, only on the sides. He knew me, knew how this would melt me, and I moaned in ecstasy. His teasing smirk told me that he knew he had me, all of me, there and then. I squirmed in pleasure, and he directed me towards Gabriel's cock, which was now ready for more pleasure.

Gabriel had to hold on to the shelf to his right for stability. Tristan licked my juices. Amused, he said, "Mmm ... you smell so good. I bet she feels good too, 'eh Gabriel?" Gabriel, getting his cock sucked off, his eyes closed, could only muster an open-mouthed, "Ahha." I stopped sucking and smiled. Tristan quickly positioned himself behind me since I was on all fours. In doggy style, he could pound me and hit all the right spots. Giving head was so much easier this way – the pounding was working for us all. They high-fived each other in action, a move better known as the Eiffel Tower*, or what I liked to call "going to Paris." That night, I went to Paris, or our "version" of it, with me the common denominator while they both switched on and off.

Jay was watching from the couch. He actually got water for Gabriel and Tristan and poured it into their mouths. I laughed at how we didn't miss a beat, not even when it came to getting hydrated. We decided to take a break, laughed, and yelled, "And 'scene'!" Jay said, "That was hot!" I thanked him even though I was still naked and panting. Gabriel said my tongue had moves and so did my vaginal walls. I had been playing with his dick, tensing inside. He loved it, and if it hadn't been for the drugs, he would have cum over five times by now.

Gabriel and Tristan decided to give each other water through a straw while the other was fucking me. It was 5:55 am, time for a new play position. We called it "The London Bridge"*, me on the bottom, one guy fucking me on top, another guy holding my legs up by my feet for better positioning, one with more stimulation and depth. He could also move my legs around to give the other guy a different feel, and I could play with the dick of the guy holding my feet up. They both switched on and off in our newfound position. Loving the teamwork and the guys' compliments, I was in awe, just looking at how everything seemed to happen so seamlessly that night. More sass was to follow our endless endeavours and fruitful wet lips begging to dive deeper.

Jay, our third guy, finally came in to play. He had been having fun jerking himself off while watching all the sights and sounds. His butch, oversized muscles made his shirt tight, defining his figure. Everything on him was muscled. Smiling and looking at me, he said, "I don't know if she can handle it." I looked back at him in challenge mode and knew I could handle it. I asked Tristan if it was ok. He said, "Of course," gleaming with excitement. And so there were, three wise men, tagging each other in, taking breaks in between, and me getting pleased every second with no breaks. Everybody had condoms on, lots of lube inside for easy gliding so all parties would be more satisfied. They would take turns, petting me, groping me, me sucking them off, them pounding me from the back or from the top, switching it up, and tossing my slim figure around.

I loved it. I like it a little rough, too. I felt sexy, wanted, in charge. I was in awe. The night continued till our limbs couldn't take it anymore. Finally, we realized how late it was and how parched I was. I finally had to stop because my pussy was sore—but in a good, satisfied way. Also, there was my back pain. I looked at the time and laughed. It was 7:30 am and getting light out as we drove back, only for one more go at sensual sex to top off the night, this one between me and my lover, Tristan. We had thought we had no juice left … one always has some stored for sex.

## The Lessons

While it may seem like every chapter has to have a dilemma, we are nearing the end, and the "kinks" (no pun intended) are starting to smooth, making way for more extravagant play, the kind where "The Vixen" can step in and own her ground.

While I am not one to say drugs are a good idea, I will say it is a good idea to always get them tested if you do ever end up trying them. Also, don't ever do them alone; always do them with people you trust. Do your research, and never do them just because someone asked you to or suggested it, or if they were just given to you, so "why not."

I have been drugged before, and it is not fun. It wasn't even at a party. I was with my friends, going houseboating, and we all went to another person's boat, someone we had just met, because his friend was a DJ spinning tunes. He offered me a drink. I took it. It tasted funny, and when I told my friend, he swatted it out of my hand. Moments later, I was in and out of consciousness. My friend threw me over his arm, fireman style, whistled loud, and shouted at everyone to leave now. Needless to say, he had saved me. I had only had a sip or two. There were others on that boat full of predators who drugged women so they could do who knows what to them. I am happy to say that they didn't get that chance with me, and I am thankful every day for my friend who saved me. I thought it was a simple drink. Do NOT accept any drinks that you didn't see poured, and inspect the bottle if you are not at an establishment. I have also seen bottles spiked. It's better to be safe, seen, and secure than to do something stupid because it was fun, fast, and easy. Stay safe out there.

In the scenes above, we had a full night of wonderful fun, new experiences, and three men with one woman (MMMF, why hello!). This was something that was possible within our dynamic, something that was a definite kink for Tristan. He described it to me as showing me off by allowing a select few—with everyone's consent—to have a taste of what he gets all the time. Watching me from the sidelines, seeing the pleasure rise turns him on. He wants to go first and last. It's not for everyone, but it's for more than you'd think. Over the years, his kink has flourished, twisted, turned, been something to navigate, and even more so, had its ups and downs. However, that's the glory of it—things can change, check-ins are important, and our relationship comes first.

As you read, one more kink of mine revealed itself—breath play or sexual/erotic asphyxiation. This form of play must be talked about ahead of time and must really be done in a safe manner. That said, the way the blood flow is restricted, OMG, intensifies my sex, helping me really zone in on the awareness of how pleasurable and intense my orgasms can be. Breath play is not for everyone, but it is for this little Vixen.

Seeing how well he shut down something I didn't want, communicating with just a look, is what happens when you are blissfully in sync. It's not always perfect—nothing is. I hope this gives you more insight into what can be possible for you or enlightens you to venture towards something you may have wanted to try in a safe, consensual way, something that will make you thrive. Sometimes, just talking about it is all that is needed too and that's fun in and of itself.

# Glossary

*Breath Play*: This type of play seeks to restrict someone's breathing for the purpose of pleasure.

*Compersion*: This quality is well known in the lifestyle or BDSM/kink community. The opposite of jealousy, compersion allows you to experience pleasure from seeing your partner get pleasure.

*Cuckolding*: With this kink, your partner loves watching you have sex with another person. Seeing you get pleasure, knowing they're going to get it as well, turns them on. Cuckolding is done of course with the consent of all parties involved. And it is not as uncommon as you would think.

*Eiffel Tower / Going to Paris*: In this instance, we did MMF (two males and one female). The woman is on all fours and in between the two guys. She sucks one of the guys off while the other one pounds her from behind, then the two guys high-five. Without the high-fives, apparently, this position is called a *split roast*, which isn't a very sexy name, but comes from the view of the person in the middle being "skewered." Needless to say, thank God for high-fives!

*G-spot*: This area is located two to three inches inside a woman's vagina, usually up the front of the vaginal wall, between the vaginal opening and the urethra. You know you have hit the "spot" when you feel a soft, squishy, almost sponge-like texture. This well-known spot got its "G" from a German gynecologist named Ernest Gräfenberg in 1981.

*Impact Play*: This is a type of play that involves using toys or instruments for pain that is pleasurable. It can be a huge turn-on, and consent, of course, is a must.

*The London Bridge*: This position is a combination of the superhero, the asteroid, and the bridge. The woman is on her back, her legs pointing towards the ceiling, and a guy pounds her between the legs, while another holds her legs (could be one or two people). The woman or the guy or guys holding her legs is/are free to fondle any of the others, whatever everyone is up for.

*Orgasmic Control*: This practice involves controlling yourself from orgasming by stopping or slowing down, usually with breathing, and then bringing yourself back to the peak.

*Sensual Play*: This form of erotic pleasure makes you horny with light touch/massaging. "Sensual" is one of five erotic blueprints founded by a somatic sexologist, Jaiya. The other erotic blueprints are: energetic, sexual, kinky, and shapeshifter. This idea is similar to that of the five love languages**, but for intimacy and pleasure.

*Sexual/Erotic Asphyxiation or Breath Play*: This sexual practice is a kind of breath play in which one intentionally restricts their or their partner's oxygen by chocking, hanging, or other means. Erotic asphyxiation is a BDSM term under the umbrella term of "breath play." This kind of play can be dangerous so be mindful; there have been deaths related to erotic asphyxiation.

*Squirting*: During orgasm/ejaculation, a woman can expel fluid. Some say it is a deep release, almost as if they've peed; some report it as an overflow of fluid; and some don't even know what happened until it did. Don't be discouraged; not everyone can squirt, and that's ok. Also, squirting can be messy so better have lots of towels on board.

*The Sex Show*: This "upscale" adult playground is dedicated to enhancing the lifestyle, encouraging romance, personal betterment, and all things taboo. This is usually accomplished through demonstrations, intimacy trinkets, promoting sex workers, pole dancing, kink, introductions to BDSM, prizes, and art.

# 18

# THE VIXEN'S NIGHT OF XXXMAS PLAY

⁓This is a night of wonder, exploration, and delight. After a long time of figuring out what I like, love, and desire, I finally knew: setting the scene, creating the atmosphere, and connecting like-minded people for freedom of exploration. It was a calling I embodied. I love the holidays, and what's better than making the holidays less stressful with a full-on, sex-positive, kinky, sexy Santa play party. Yo-ho-ho, you sexy sluts! Get your whips out and your open minds on. It was time to adventure and open our house up to selected individuals for a sexy private party for sinners and saints.⁓

*I*t was a mansion of a house, full of wonder and exploration. There were rooms with different themes and more, and Tristan and I were in a great spot in our relationship. We had nipped a lot of things in the bud, and through those experiences, we continued to grow together. This story details a night of awe, a night to let go and more so, a night filled with friends we adore. This was our XXXmas party, come one, come all. Bring your spunk but not your funk. This is where differences were left at the door, the ego/the shadow/the mind is shed. This is where communication is key, and consent is a must. Here you are to embrace a "less is more" approach and let the naughty little elves frolic. People come dressed up to dress down and play all around. Come with an open mind and open heart. No cameras, no phones; fight club rule number one, "You don't talk about fight club," meaning anyone invited was not to talk about the party to others. This is critical to making sure a party stays private, and even more so, helps keep others' intimate lives private as well. Most in attendance were high profile businesspeople who knew how to have a good time, even if nothing happens.

Welcome to the play party.

The house was bright with fun and flare and lights of delight. The décor was on point, and the DJ was spinning tunes, including dirty Santa songs; the dance floor was lit up with lights that flickered to the beat, and Christmas decorations adorned the windows and surroundings. The three fireplaces were fired up to max, bringing a hot sizzle to the cool winter night. Let us slay that sleigh all the way down low. For easing muscles and minds, the hot tub was on full blast, and the pool was heated, both steaming the cool air into mist. Fire pits were lined up in a row for flow along the walkway, tents stationed over them for cover and privacy, trapping the heat for chats. Seats, throw blankets, and onesies for keeping warm and cozy throughout the night were plentiful inside the tents as well. Reindeer, bad Santas, Santa's elves, Miss Naughty Clause, dirty Santas, and everything in between—you name it! Along the side, of course, BDSM** accessories and kink tantalized the eyes. Santa had a paddle, an elf had restraints, and ooh, boy was there anything and everything.

Let's set the atmosphere a bit more …

Welcome to the mansion of sinners and saints. Upon entry, the staircase spirals downward as if it has a story all its own to tell. Near the entrance, on the right, there is a chill room full of white leather La-Z-Boy couches against the walls, fluffy blankets on the floor in the middle, and a Christmas tree with our very own, very talented photographer. Props and décor match the roaring fireplace (one of many!). A snowy light glistened in the white ceiling, making this the cuddle room for all.

Next, moving clockwise, you'll find the grand dining room for eats and treats to ease your eyes and your tummies. Here anyone can relax from the noise and replenish their soul. Exiting into the open-concept kitchen, everyone congregates, drinking and being merry before spilling into a nook and coming upon the dance floor. The hall then leads towards the bathrooms, then full circle back to the spiral stairs. Every inch of the place is decorated with lights, knick-knacks, stickers, candies, and more. Two turkeys, plus the fixings, are surrounded by all the other Xmas-themed potluck offerings, all deliciously delightful food.

Tiptoeing along up the stairs, you'll find four rooms for the sinners, the saints, and the all. The saints' room is lined with white lights and white, lavish, snowy décor. Next to the bed and the couch, there is a station with condoms, lube, and towels. The door can be shut for privacy and more, along with a sign that reads "Closed for privacy" on one side and "Open for viewing" on the other. Newbies or shy guests can delight and play** without being fully exposed.

The next room is all red, with a bed and a leather couch for viewing. The door to this room can be shut as well, but it symbolizes one step closer to becoming a full sinner on Santa's naughty list. The next room holds the orgy bed, which is king size, and a lovely, jackhammering Sybian machine** with a dial for speed. The light is red as well, the whole room naughtier than the saints' room.

The last room is where the sinners are. The door is wide open, a hole where the knob used to be. It was made for exploring, igniting, and tantalizing the senses. Decorated with red lights, tea lights line the floor, and a St. Andrew's cross** in one corner. Hanging on the wall next to it are props and tools for play. There are all kinds of rope, hand cuffs, floggers**, paddles for warming up, and a stripper pole directly under a red spotlight, ever so forgiving. The king size bed is in the middle and against the wall, red leather fitted tops available for a quick change to promote cleanliness. There is also a table filled with condoms, cleaning supplies, lube, and mints. The queen size bed is outfitted the same way, complete with its own set of side tables and goodie baskets. There is also a pyramid of rolled white towels for easy cleaning up afterward, with a bin underneath for ease of disposal—thank goodness.

A sex swing hangs from the ceiling, its companion a mirror for watching every little thing. I have personally used it myself, enjoying a little katoptronophilia*. In the middle of this huge room, there is a massage table for teasing, seducing, play, and more. Coconut oil can be found underneath, for easy flow of touch. For the audience, voyeurs, and curious minds, stools are spread about, along with a couch on which to relax and enjoy the show. This is the sinners' room. It is always in full swing, and the scenes are always changing.

*Welcome to the play party, I hope you cum again*, I say to myself with a grin and wink.


This was our sanctuary, our Garden of Eden, and our event of the year for the wild, sexy ones whose desires, fantasies, and lustful sins would be welcomed upon request and with consent.

After greetings, laughter, pouring drinks, clothing changes, and photo op moments, the night was finally getting into the groove: the music sexier, the house fuller, naughtiness frolicking about. In the "chill" room, tons of people were relaxing, chatting, and enjoying the atmosphere, and *each other*. Fondling and grinding could be seen throughout.

I stepped into the dining room to see people eating, relaxing, chatting, and laughing. Someone called out, "HEY! HEY, Z!" I turned around to be delighted by a man with a killer smile and jet-black hair, dashing blue eyes glimmering at me. When I looked at him, he looked me up and down, bit his lower lip, and leaned back in his chair. Flushing, I smiled and asked, "Sup?" He beamed and said, "Nothing. I just wanted to see all of you, Zara." I raised my eyebrows at him. It felt like a moment went by where we didn't break eye contact. I was in lustful shock, trying to figure out what to say—a witty comeback or something flirty, but all I said was, "Well, here ya go," and ran off.

His gaze had flustered me, as well as his intensity and the "take me" energy I was feeling towards his masculinity. I played with the idea in my head, but my girlfriend Brooklyn grabbed my arm and asked me to get a drink with her. We eyed each other, knowing we needed a little pick-me-up after eating and expelling energy hosting and setting up. Gleefully, we got some energy pills and ground them up in the upstairs bathroom together. That's what we needed and would be needing throughout the night, as well as check-ins with each other. She is my Master** after all, and she is amazing at knowing me and knowing what I need. We have a soul-deep, past-life type of connection that fills us every time we are together.

Brooklyn and I had met through Tristan and instantly took a liking to each other. I just felt safe with her, like she would conquer the world for me and back me up anywhere, anytime! She has a blunt attitude and does not shy away from problems or concerns; she goes full throttle, bulldozing through, completely transparent. I absolutely adore this woman. Through our ups and downs, we have always been there for each other, or communicated why in those rare moments we could not be. It is the friendship of all friendships; she is my soulmate and my Master. The dynamic between us is very beautiful. I just naturally submit to her, and her love towards me is naturally dominant. Don't get me wrong, we did toy with the idea of switching**. We tried, hated it, and never went back. Me trying to dominate her didn't feel right; it was awkward and uncomfortable. Blah! (Insert: image of me shaking my body to rid myself of the thought, like a dog shaking water out of its fur.) My Master is my master for a reason, and I trust her infinitely. She is also hilarious and full of energy, both qualities I missed in my life after my accident a while back.

After indulging in each other's company and laughing our asses off about anything and everything, silly as we were, we made our way out of the bathroom, ready for more. We were instantly blanketed with body heat from the pool of sensual people as well the vibration of the beats. I was about to go socialize when I got stopped by my lover, Tristan. He had been wondering where I was and if he could take me away for a moment. He held me in his arms, smirking, lust and wonder glistening from his husky, blue-grey eyes. I nodded, and he led me into our bedroom. I was thrilled; we love to have our time first before anyone else's, and we love to be each other's last at the end of the night. This was our way, our connection. Hand in hand, he led me towards to bed, which was right above the thundering speakers below, and kissed me passionately. I grabbed his ass … *Mmm* … his ass was oh-my-god, like a Greek god's ass—plump, muscular, and round—one I was always down to bite.

We quickly became heated and shed our clothes in desperation and passion, all while kissing each other in between each piece, revealing more skin. (I can't even tell you how hot, how Taoistic, how in sync our polarity** is.) Devouring each other's tongues, he threw me on the bed, which got my juices flowing even more. He started crawling on top of my naked body, gently kissing up my legs, checking in between and testing to make sure I was ready for him by teasing me into wanting more. I moaned and trembled for him. He smiled and said, "Damn, you're wet," before licking my swollen clit with one long glide upwards. Then he moved towards me, half his weight on me, and penetrated me all the way. My body squirmed with pleasure, and I inhaled as he thrusted in. Listening to the music, I wanted all of him inside of me. His rhythm had impetus and momentum, and then BAM, the door flung open, and there was Brooklyn.

"Oh! There you are, haha! Damn, that's hot. Want pictures?" she laughed. Tristan said, "Oh-my-god, Brooklyn. Give us a second." She remarked with a smart-ass comment, "A second ... really?!" I laughed, Tristan still inside me, and said, "Let us finish! We will be down soon ..." Then the door thudded closed again. Laughing and starry-eyed, we continued, fulfilling our longing—for the moment. Throughout the night, other people had also needed things; my energy was vibing—thank God we had this moment now.

After we got dressed and noticed how hot we were, it was game on ... or should I say ... "Party on." As we progressed down the staircase, a massage train started to form. I went along with it. Ares, the black-haired, blue-eyed babe, invited me to sit in front of him for a back rub. I looked at Tristan, and he nodded in excitement. His kink**, well, as you re-call, was watching me get noticed, touched, fucked, or played with by other guys. Go figure. It was a dominance thing and a sexy as hell thing as well. He knew I wouldn't be crossing any lines. I sat down. Once I did, more and more people joined in until there was a 35-person massage train fondling, rubbing, kissing, touching, and caressing. Oh-my-fucking-god, HOTNESS! And I was part of it, laughing at the sheer openness and how everyone assembling just kinda happened.

All the touching amplified my sex. Ares whispered in my ear, "I'm glad you're in front of me, so you can't see what I'll be doing. You'll only be able to feel the sensations of my touch." His deep voice and the whispered warmth of those fucking words caused shivers to run down my body. Damn, he had me wanting. He moved closer and told me to please tell him if he did anything I was not ok with. I was choked up with the pure ecstasy of his beauty and praise, so I just nodded. He started in on me, and I started on the lovely, vibrant woman in front of me after I'd asked her if there was anything she didn't want me to touch. She said nope. As I kept going on her, Ares continued on me, slowing working his way to my neck, then my lower back, and then even lower, to my butt. His hands never left my body unless to position my hair out of the way. *This is epic*, I thought.

Every so often, he would breathe in or nibble my ear, leading me back into his hands. I had to remember I was massaging too.

Tristan came back, beaming as he gave me a thumbs-up, and told me to stay and enjoy myself while he hosted and socialized. I was in awe. Ares slowly moved in towards my side, then inward towards my lower abdomen, all while motioning me into his clearly erect dick. I moved in sync with him, letting out sounds of pleasurable breath, closing my eyes, inviting his sexual play. Since we were in the midst of a massage train, I opened my eyes to see everyone getting friskier and friskier, some getting penetrated, others nibbling on nipples. I was almost innocent compared to the others. I reminded myself to lean towards the woman in front of me, making sure to pump my ass back towards Ares so he could glide with me.

The woman loved my touch, and even more so, she loved how the energy invited everyone to be in the moment. I caressed her boobs and nibbled her ear, and she wiggled her bubble butt with excitement. Through my underwear, Ares was sliding his finger along my throbbing clit, massaging it while my ass was still up. I was giving more attention to the woman in front, but I gently wiggled my hips, inviting him for more. Getting to massage the woman and bite her shoulder brought me pleasure. She kept giggling, "Yes." I slowly leaned back again and pumped my back towards Ares. He kissed my pussy right before I plopped my ass back down on the stairs and right against his rock-hard cock again, slowly increasing the pressure. I was blushing and getting higher with each touch and all the sounds and play in action. He moved in towards my boobs and played with my nipples, clamping them between his fingers and massaging them. I jolted with pleasure, breathing heavy to match. He rubbed his lips along my neck, and I was hooked. I knew I need to move now, or I'd be sucked in. I let it go on for a few more moments before leaning back to thank him. In reply, he winked and gave me a "no, thank YOU, it was my pleasure," smile with his gorgeous straight teeth. I thanked the woman in front before slipping out of there. She was hot and heavy from getting pleased in two directions. The line was starting to disperse but kept going for a little while longer.

When I went into the kitchen, Tristan greeted me and told me to give him the details. It was a turn-on for him, so I obeyed and whispered a few things in his ear. I saw his dick get hard as he imagined what I'd been doing. He grabbed his cock as it throbbed from hearing my story and said, "Look how my body responds to you." I bit my lower lip to show my enjoyment. He beamed at me and said, "If you want to do anything else with someone, let me know. I'm good!" I smiled and said, "Thanks, but I want to dance and drink." We had a few shots of tequila together, and I went off dancing while Tristan stood by. Every so often, he would look at me, see my enjoyment and eye me up while I danced seductively on the dance floor. Every so often, the DJ would give us a helicopter*, and the dance floor would roar with amusement.

As more people arrived, the place got hotter, and so did the attire. Barely-there lingerie—everything everywhere was delightful to watch. As you know, watching is one of my things. I love seeing people experience pure pleasure and enjoyment—being open and free and able to express and undress with ease and without obligation. This is why consent culture is so important and where it comes into play. Just because I am expressing my sexual energy, my desire to dress sexy, and my freedom to be nude does not mean you can touch me or I can touch you.

*You may gaze gently but every hold tight till an ask is be yonder told.*

Everyone was getting frisky on the dance floor, and I wanted to just frolic around and say hi. I left as things started getting dirtier and hotter. I told Tristan I was going to wander downstairs. We had agreed we wouldn't go in the play rooms upstairs without each other—that was our *thang*. Tristan nodded happily and grabbed my ass as I swayed by in my red lace bra and red garter belt with white fluffy cuffs and a black G-string to match. The garter wasn't attached to anything, but I had matching thigh-high stockings, white and red, and a nice Santa hat that I would switch out for reindeer antlers later.

My fluttery fake lashes were inviting, pulling others in my direction. Swiftly, I went into the lounge room where one of my buddies was. We lay down and watched the ceiling glisten majestically. Everyone there was in cuddle-puddle heaven or doing even more than that … I might have made it too comfortable for people to want to stay in. After complimenting each other and catching up, the hour flew by. We looked around, and the room had become an orgy haven, as if we were in Greek or Roman mythological times. Oops! I am not one to shame or blame people in their element, so I just stood up to remind people that they could go upstairs for that kind of fun and to help move them in that direction. *That's a win*, I said in my head. Before venturing onward and grabbing a water along the way, I turned to my friend and thanked them for coming and for catching up. I had needed that.

Brooklyn and I were running around, restocking the rooms, making sure people were ok. We restarted and refilled the hot tub. In general, we were doing everything anyone asked for—be it ice, a Band-Aid, a whip, a twirl, or to clean up a spill or show someone where to find something. It was exhausting and exciting at the same time. Master and I only had to nod or grunt or even just look at each other to know what was needed. We were in our element.

After making sure everything was handled, we looked around. The place was bumping, 150 guests circulating, having loads of fun. We kicked four people out, warned two others, and had to help one who was having a bad trip. Since she was sitting in the corner, looking into space, I was grateful I found her. I got her some cold water, found her man, and she was good to go. I am happy to be able to create such a wonderful atmosphere full of sex-positivity**, community, and safety. As I was beaming and smiling at these thoughts, Brooklyn pulled me upstairs towards the bathroom again.

She quickly closed the door and went, "Whee!!!!" I started laughing my ass off, falling to the ground. I was in awe of the purity and the vibes she was putting out … Then it hit me, *It is bloody hot up here, and wow, does that make you higher! Oh no, now into the giggles we go* … We spent another 45 minutes laughing on the floor, abs hurting, eyes watering, giggling up a storm … till Tristan walked in and said, "There you are!" In excitement, I hugged and kissed him, telling him to come in and join us for a bit. "Shit, it's hot in here," he said. "You guys need to take a break. Let me help." Brooklyn and I nodded at Tristan and got up, upping our energy once more (insert: Mario going from small to full-size sound). Brooklyn went tumbling downstairs, her feet in super speed mode, to frolic and socialize once more, and Tristan and I started making our way to the playrooms, watching the scenes as we came upon them.

Mallory was getting double penetrated by the jack hammer dildo and her significant other. Behind them, a threesome MWW* was happening on the king size bed. The juicy noises were flourishing. Tristan and I smiled and said hi to everyone. We fondled each other while watching others … sooo heavenly. He felt me up between my thighs and kissed my neck. I grabbed his ass and teased his cock. Mallory piped up and said, "Well, I tried it …" Her partner turned the knob, and she went, "Ooh … ok, let's give it another chance." They smiled and kissed with delight. Tristan and I looked at each other and moved towards the saint room, which was in use, unfortunately and fortunately, according to the closed door and the sign. We moved on to the other single red room where the DJ was making a woman squirt** for the first time ever. She was howling with pleasure and curiosity about the unknown. We sat against the couch as another couple watched them on the bed, riding each other, her on top and loving it. He was grabbing her ass, and every so often, he would glance over to take in the juicy views and moans of others. It was a lovely scene**; they were communicating throughout, and she was nervous since she had never done it before. She was unsure if she had to pee or squirt. The DJ told her to relax into the pleasure sensation.

Tristan and I watched with wonder and delight, both in awe at how we had created this, how we got to have this when most people don't get to explore it in their life. After the scene climaxed, towels started flying, and there was more fondling. We made our way to the bigger room with the full BDSM-theme, kink, sex swing, and more—where the sinners were. The room was all red, glowing with candles, and wide open. It was hot in that room; on the king size bed, two couples were going at it. The queen size bed was occupied by a woman with luscious red hair devouring two men, one going down on her, all while she still had her heels on. Another couple watched it all from the sex swing and fondled each other. On the St. Andrew's cross, a playmate was tied up and getting punished—licked, flogged, and spanked. To increase her wonder and excitement, and to let her sensations run wild, she was blindfolded with a silk black tie. Clothes were flung everywhere, and the red lighting gave each scene a seductive glow. The couch was full. People were spilling onto the ground, cuddling and watching the scenes while chatting or just rubbing each other lightly. All enjoyed the sights, sounds, and heat of the room. Throughout the night, all the rooms would be busy with different scenes.

Tristan and I plopped down in the cuddle-puddle on the floor. Everyone beamed at us and said hi. Wowza, it was hot, steamy, and making me a tad frisky. I was joking around and spouting off direction to a couple I knew well. Everyone, including the guy, started laughing, and the woman giggled, "Z! Come on, I had a rhythm." She signaled for me to zip my mouth shut.

Tristan and I started getting hot and bothered, so I seductively went down on him. His dick was thick and just the right size for making me squirm while sucking him off. I looked up at him every so often since he liked that. He massaged my head, and I twirled my tongue around his shaft, teasing his tip. I could feel his veins filling more, the pulse, the pump, harder and harder, till he grabbed my head and said, "Fuck! I need to fuck you!" I spun around on command. He leaned in to give everyone a front row seat, thrusting as I gulped with pleasure and excitement. His hardness made me bite down on my hand. He was fully erect and throbbing. My sex was longing, and a few more minutes in, I saw the bed was free now,

so I stopped and threw him down on the queen. I placed his cock
in my hand, gave him a lick, and submerged his shaft in my wet
pussy. My red bed was getting fuller with every minute that went
by; my knees were on the outskirts, pressing him down to hold my
stance. I rode him with pleasure and ease, lustfully gliding my hips
up and in towards him, making myself moan more. He pulled me
in to kiss him and threw me on my back so he could fuck me. And
he fucked me good. He wanted me, needed me, and I could feel it
coming from every cell of his body. I gripped his sides to pull him
closer to me. He gripped my throat for a few moments to tell me
who he was—my Sir**. I moaned, wanting more, needing more. I
was shaking. I closed my eyes, letting the lust engulf me. We stopped
and breathed deeply, heavily, both sweaty, kissing passionately as if
it were our last. We smiled at each other and took a break on both
our backs. One person piped up, "Damn! That was hot!" I laughed.
I had forgotten that we were the scene—the entertainment. Lots
of people had been watching the show, enjoying the view and the
tantalizing tease.

Holding hands, together we stumbled out after having again
gotten dressed (-ish). Even though we were parched, we smiled at
everyone saying "Thank you" or offering prayer hands and thumbs-up
gestures. Our friends always cheered people on no matter what,
making sure they felt seen and appreciated. We made our way to the
bathroom to clean up a bit and splash water on our faces. I touched
up my makeup, and we went downstairs again for more water,
nourishment, and refreshments, all while glowing with pleasure.

Tristan and I were passionate, delicately in love, and driven
for each other. Even the way we looked at each other made my
body quiver; I would get all warm and fuzzy inside. The kids (Did
I mention Tristan has two kids?) were staying with friends for the
weekend, and this knowledge just made our sense of freedom and
play even more so. The aftermath, scavenger hunts, and surprises
left behind after tonight would not be so kid friendly, however, to
say the least. As I was passing, Tristan reached for me and swung

me around to plant a wonderful kiss on my mouth, a kiss full of energy, mischief, and lust. I was hooked. He had me … all of me. I opened my eyes at the end of our kiss to be further devoured by his essence and dominant presence. In each other's arms, we drew others' attention with the sheer energy emanating from our core.

The house was full, everything was getting used, and scenes ebbed and flowed with the night's tides. The house was nay so quiet as a mouse, to say the least; however, it was pure bliss.

After running around during another round of "Is there anything that needs a topping or encouraging?", I ended up back in the bathroom with my great friend, my Master and safe human, giggling all over the floor once more. Tristan again found us, and this time, he was over the moon and wanted to play. Brooklyn got her play bag out, and BAM, small dildo for the win. Tristan did not want that. "Anything but," he said. I told him it was unfair that someone else had gotten the privilege, and I hadn't. This somehow swayed him, and he hesitantly agreed. I told him he could trust me and to just speak up if it got too much. I would go slow, use lots of lube, and talk to him gently, *teeheehee*. I was in heaven. My man trusted me enough to go inside him with the smallest dildo we had, attached to my harness. What color you might ask? Purple!

Brooklyn gave us pointers. It was great. He was nervous but took it like a champ. I told him that the worst thing he could do for himself was tense and tighten up because it could become more painful. With that in mind, he spread his cheeks and away we went! Lubed up and breathing deeply to relax, I went slowly and gently. He actually relaxed and wasn't as bad as before, when he'd had a killer experience with a Dominatrix** that plowed into him and was not the best; she had had her way with him, and it was not so gentle. I was happy he trusted me for this and happy to tell him I would never do it again unless he asked. He replied that he wouldn't, but that it was great to give me his last experience. Guys have an erotic zone there, and so do women; however, not all do, so I only did it for a little bit and pulled out. He was happy when I stopped and happy that it wasn't like the last time. Just having the experience made me smile ear to ear, and I gave him a towel to clean up. It was fun, and now on to the next!

Brooklyn said, "Ok, well, that was hot. I'm going to go and check in." She went speeding towards the door in her lingerie to go find her partner. Tristan got off the bed and started cleaning up. I asked if he'd had a rim job* before. He was hesitant and unsure; he said probably once. I confirmed he was clean and asked if I could. Unfortunately, he had experienced trauma there, so I did not push, but he allowed me to, and I was gentle once again. I told him to tell me to stop for any reason at all. He got back on the bed, face down, and I slowly kissed his legs and inner thighs before I dove in and started licking and playing. I had never done it either. I like having firsts, especially with my Sir, my lover, my beloved. He was high, so he actually moaned and said, "That feels good," and, "I like what you're doing," while I navigated. Normally, he wasn't expressive, but he was now. I was indulging and enjoying the experience, and I would totally do it again if he allowed me to or wanted it (of course as long as he cleaned and maybe trimmed beforehand). I kept teasing, and I tongue-fucked him a bit all the while licking him up. I only did it for a little while, until he flipped around, wanting me. I paused and went to go use mouthwash.

When I came back, he grabbed me full force, pulled me down, and proceeded to go down on me. OMG, was he excited to do so, claiming me with each flick and glide of his tongue, engorging my pink vulva to intensity. He knew how to pleasure me fully, licking me softly, lightly even though he had the power to do what he wished. I was in pure surrender. My hips went with the motion, his hands on both sides of them ... *Holy ... Ooh my ... Yes ...* I repeated over and over, moaning louder till I clenched. He knew to grab my throat a bit to make me cum harder. I love that he knows me. I grabbed the sheets and arched my back, holding my breath till I burst with pure

ecstasy, breathing out a huge, "OOOoooo ahhhhhhmmmmmm …"
Slowly, he slid up to claim what was rightfully his. We smiled and
gazed at each other with pure infatuation. I was his and he was mine.
He had missed me passionately and so glided his erect cock into my
primed pussy. He was gentle as I inhaled quickly when he started
penetrating me. Soon, my wet sex lubed up his shaft. He increased
the rhythm, going faster. It quickly got heated, and I grabbed him,
scratching only slightly. I longed to mark my territory. I was in my
primal mode, my moment, my body clinging to him, needing him to
go deeper. He went in and out in succulent movements, permeating
my wholeness. We breathed each other's breath in a sensational,
tantric flow. I closed my eyes to feel him fully. He pulsated inside of
me, getting harder and ready to blow. I clenched my pelvic floor, and
he let out a pure, shallow breath, the kind that showed he had tried
to ride the edge** but couldn't hold. He pulled out and released with
an *ahhh* … all over my front. I smiled in satisfaction, not because he
had cum, but because I had driven him wild—wild enough that he
couldn't hold it anymore.

After a quick rinse and clean up, we had to check in, and holy
hotness, the place was heated with bodies, friction, sensualness,
sexiness, lust, and sooo much blissful yumminess. We made our way
towards the red room so we could just watch. It was open, but Rick
came straight up to me and said, "Hey, I have been looking for you!
I washed my hands and my mouth!" He was an epic lover, attuned,
and he had a foot fetish**. He loved my feet and knew how to suck
them off in such a way that made me realize he had skills. I looked
at him with pure delight (I am a tad germophobic), but I was also
exhausted. I had to tell Rick, "Rain check? Gotta replenish." With
compassion, he put his hands up and said, "No problem, you know
where I'll be." He smirked and gave me a big, squeezing hug. Tristan
was behind me, and he said, "That was hot." I replied, "Down, tiger.
Let's chill for a bit."

In the red room, someone was getting flogged on the St.
Andrew's cross, and an audience was watching a consensual gang

bang. I smiled at Tristan and whispered, "I think this was the couple whose husband announced downstairs, 'I can't please my wife alone. Please help, guys. Help me please my wife. Let's meet upstairs in half an hour.'" Tristan's head went back in blissful shock, and he said, "Wow, ok, let's see this." I was in his arms, leaning on the couch, the show right in front of us.

One of Tristan's fantasies was for me to get gang banged. It wasn't my fantasy, but I enjoyed how turned on he got, how it was something he liked to watch and maybe partake in. With a grin, he would always say to me, "As long as I'm last." It was almost as if his fantasy went back to primal times when the guy with the bigger head on his dick would win by fucking the woman last and taking out any other guy's semen. To me, it was a dominant thing, but he says he likes to show me off by sharing what he has and teasing others in the process. It gets him off; it's his kinky side, his fantasy, his porn. I think I might one day do this for him, even though I don't want to since it does not interest me. The thrill in Tristan's eyes and the adventure it would bring—he would be forever mine and me forever his. The parameters would be vital; the guys would have to be people I trusted, who would never talk about it or bring it up again ever. I used to be one of those people—I found out—who fucks and chucks*. Basically, I liked having a consensual experience and then never seeing them again; just let it be. I wouldn't even talk about the experience again unless my partner wanted to for fun, but that's it. I didn't want the other person in my life because I had someone in my life already; more would be too complicated. Another thing: the other guys would have to be shooting blanks, meaning no sperm swimmers present. I do not want there to be any possibility of me getting pregnant.

In the show in front of us, guy after guy had a go with the guy's wife, and she loved how rough, how hard, and how pushy the guys were. The audience grew and grew at the scene, intrigued and in awe of what was transpiring. Every few minutes, another guy would get in line and rub himself with excitement. The woman on the bed said, "Next," while her husband watched her taking it, gorging on the yeses and telling her that she liked it. This was a dynamic I'd usually only seen on a screen. I was quiet, alternating between looking at Tristan and back at the scene. He was excited, whispering in my ear, "You could do better!" I blushed. The vibrant woman before us was taking a beating. She loved getting her ass beaten with a wooden paddle till she bruised black. After numerous men got sucked, fucked, and devoured by her luscious vibes, the show was over and clean up and aftercare** were underway. Her man gave it to her, rubbing her ass, holding her, kissing her, and telling her how hot she was, while the other men cleaned up as if they were her slaves in a hot, tropical climate.

Tristan and I ventured downstairs to dance and socialize, and then we realized it was 4 am. We were amazed and in awe of how the night had gone. Around 2 am, half the people had already left in party buses towards Ontario, but the long haulers were carrying on the night as they usually did. Tristan was indulging his extroverted side with social surface talk as I got my dance on to the Nuance-brand speakers, vibing on the dance floor. The music was pure and clean; tech beats were my jam throughout the night. Brooklyn skipped over to me, and we started dancing hard and giggling. She'd had sex and was glowing. I knew because I had heard her from below. She is a loud partner; her voice carries when she openly expresses her pleasure, which is ALWAYS! Fuck, I love her. Suddenly, we looked at each other and needed to up our game. What number were we on …? Who cares? Dancing for an hour had depleted us. We needed water and energy, so we popped some into our system and replenished our souls.

Tristan reminded me to go visit Rick. I agreed, and after enjoying our bubble of giggles once again, Brooklyn and I popped over to Rick, and I asked him, "You ready?" His eyes widened playfully, and he replied, "One sec. I gotta wash my hands again." I gestured for him to meet us at the top of the staircase where a lounger sat against the wall. He nodded, and I quickly got Tristan, washed my feet, and freshened up. Rick met up with me once more, and together we entered a zone that could only be called orgasmic. He told me to lie down after putting a nice, comfy towel down so there was a barrier between the carpet and me. Rick knew me, knew that I hated dirty places. From there, he began massaging my legs, and more people formed around us. Tristan started touching me, as did Brooklyn, and Rick said, "Her feet are mine. You can have the rest." I giggled. Suddenly, I had eight hands on me. Rick was caressing and teasing, licking my toes. It was heavenly. Others had tried and failed, but he just knew how. He did it with such ease and precision that fucked me hard. I kept wanting more and motioned to tell them so. The thrill of others touching me and caressing me ignited my sex.

Rick sucked my toes and licked in between them. I tried to pay attention to how, but *ohmygod*, I couldn't concentrate. His eroticism was making me go higher, heated in the moment of Shiva*and Shakti*. I was squirming. Rick hummed and kept up the sexy talk, "Ooh … she likes that," and, "Ooh … you can't get enough, can you?" I kept nodding, wanting. It was as if his tongue was penetrating my sex, without penetrating me. I was near cumming, and my breath was heavy. I didn't think I had any more left in me, but I let out a huge sigh and trembled, cumming from the sensational energy elements that had been building. I didn't know toe licking could make me cum, make me desire, and get me into a higher frequency that was heavenly. *DAMN!* I thought. I looked around. Wow, I had forgotten so many people were around, including Tristan. They commented on his and my abilities, about how it had all come about and how they had all taken part.

Robert asked if he could continue with me. He looked at Tristan, who nodded in excitement, and I agreed. Rick kissed my toes goodbye, and I hugged him from the floor and said, "Holy fuck, thank you …" Then Robert slid in, asking me if I had ever had a G-spot** orgasm. Thinking back, I had tried with different people, but nope, never. "Well, here is your lucky day. I'll guide you if you like." I was nervous and excited. He asked for towels since he didn't want everything to get wet with my juices. I piped up to say I was a gusher, not a squirter. He said, "You just haven't squirted yet then." I was gonna reply, but Brooklyn piped in, "No, not everyone is." I looked at her in gratitude. Tristan was excited, and Brooklyn decided to take a break and go back upstairs. Up there, people were forming and getting sexy all around, aroused by the show and the talent.

Robert knew me too. In a sexy voice, he whispered, "I washed my hands." I smiled and giggled. I was drifting into delicious delirium, wanting play that was sexy, sensual, and full of care. He pep-talked me about what to expect, which I had never had before. I umm'd and ok'd and nodded a lot. We came up with a double tap and a word to use that would stop the play. "Pineapple" was the word. He mentioned he would communicate little tidbits along the way. He proceeded slowly with the upward motion he had said he was going to do. He kept it up, progressing with a tad more speed. My body was filling up, feeling squirmy when Robert whispered in my ear, "You will get to a point where it's uncomfortable. Go through that. You may find a spot where you think you're gonna pee. Go through that and relax into it." I nodded, and he continued. More people surrounded us, playing around us. Some were beside me, some petting me, playing with my nipples*. Three on the lounge chair were going at it while watching me as if this was live porn helping tease them into play. I felt like a queen who was getting ready for her king, prepped and teased, horny and wet, waiting to get devoured by her king. I was in awe.

I got to the point Robert said would be uncomfortable, so I relaxed and told him so with a nod. He continued but faster. I instantly vibrated my body into harmonious pleasure; his finger played me like I was a violin. I pressed into the pressure on my abdomen, ooh-ing and ahh-ing, my nipples being played with at the same time. I let out any sound that would escape me. My high was from pleasure alone, and sex ecstasy is a thing—I was there. I was feeling orgasmic ecstasy hard. My nipples wanting more, Tristan kissing me, and Robert rapid-firing my G-spot till 45 minutes blew by, and I let out the biggest orgasm of my life. I vibrated, moaned, and gushed, still holding his hands inside me. He slowly, ever so gently moved to continue my orgasm, prolonging it into next level Atlantis. He rode my edge hard. Among the many orgasms I have had, this was my very first G-spot orgasm. I had popped my cherry, and man, was it epic. Others had helped the show along. I realized a while ago that I do get really stimulated by nipple play, and damn, it had got me into my presence, along with Tristan kissing me and being there to enjoy the moment with me. Our bond is powerful.

We slowly got up, the people around us in pure awe, feeling blessed about having experienced such a show. Tristan and I headed down the spiral stairs and into the garage where drinking and chatting was happening. I randomly found a cock ring* on top of the table, so I quickly washed it and asked Tristan to put it on. Lo and behold! I knew he wouldn't enjoy it; however, he had never worn one before, so why the fucking hell not try? He smiled and asked, "What do I do?" I talked him through it and went to my knees on the cement to put it on him. While I was down there, I sucked him off. He was happy that I was doing it in front of more people but still wasn't sure about the cock ring. To my surprise, the two guys with us chatted with him about their own experiences. My mouth was full, so I listened. I couldn't help but giggle. Tristan asked me to bend over so he could try to fuck me with the cock ring on. Needless to say, total fail. As soon as I stopped sucking him off, Tristan started to go soft. He was not enjoying the ring. He fucked me a bit, and I said, "There, you tried. You hate it, and now you know." He took it off, sighing at the sense of relief. He said thank you, and we all moved on in the wee hours of the morning. We kicked back in the chill room where lounging and pouncing was happening next to the fire. It looked like a 70's era scene, people tripping, talking, and caressing. Vavoom! After a few chats, delighting in the fresh air from outside, firepits still roaring, I made my way to the hot tub to let my body ease. I enjoyed blissful foot rubs, while giving them as well, and the early morning chats. The briskness on my face and the steam of the hot tub was a wonderful sight and feeling. The group that was left was usually my main group. They knew to bring their gear for a long night. I always had one expression: "Fuck, I have fun friends!" Awe and a smile gleamed on my face when I expressed that out loud. Brooklyn laughed, "You can say that again!"

The next day was clean-up time. The people who stayed helped. We are a community after all and take care of things respectfully. We did hire a cleaning crew, and fuck, was it disastrous, as well as fucking hilarious—a scavenger hunt for clothes, a joke on what was found in the hot tub, and more. Dirty shit was everywhere, and OMG, come on, people, you know how to put your used condoms in the garbage! They were all over! Needless to say, gloves and hand sanitizer are your friends the next day.

## The Lessons

This sex-positive environment wasn't the first or the last. We hosted countless parties to flourish and christen our relationship, including bottomless blow-glow parties (just like the name says)! Glow party and bottoms off! Shirts on; summer sizzling slip 'n slide, the adult version, slip and slide for the win. *Hello, summer fun! We get wet in more ways than one.* Tristan and I have had lots of adventures already. We are on our way to more since we are able to host, create, and navigate these parties. They were fun, exhausting, and memorable. We always tell people to come with zero expectations; be open to a variety of possibilities, be respectful of others, and make sure you own your boundaries** and respect yourself. I invite you to explore and listen to your intuition as you discover your inner vixen too.

This chapter is to focus on the fact that "shit can hit the fan" does not mean that the relationship is doomed, that you're not a great match, or that relationships should be easy. WRONG! It's work. You're talking about two people from two different backgrounds, with different beliefs, different experiences, different values, and maybe even trauma and inexperience. You both have your own way of communicating and questioning. "Listen to understand, not to respond. Be interested, not interesting." Over time, it does get easier; however, the key is to grow together and listen, see, and be heard! Integrate, accept influence, and check in with each other. Full disclaimer: I am not saying all relationships are worth going through "the shit." HELL no! If you're in a manipulative, abusive, and so forth relationship, that's not ok! Get help, get out! Talk to someone.

As for the meanings of definitions, well, different things mean different things for different people. For example, "topping" for gay men means something different than "topping" for heterosexual persons. It is best to ask if you aren't clear on what someone means. I love to ask for clarity regarding certain things, and when the other person wants to make sure they've got clarity as well, you create a safe, open atmosphere full of transparency. Can you say HOT?! That's just my sapiosexuality* coming out.

Ok, back at it … There is solid evidence now that says a 5:1 ratio is good for relationships. This framework is from John and Julia Gottman of the Gottman Institute and their 40-plus years of research and experience. A 5:1 ratio means you gotta say five nice, lean-in, appreciative things together for every "bad" or not-so-fun experience. And that's when things are going ok. When things are in the shit, well, get ready to go bigger because it then becomes a 20:1 ratio. Yes! You must each say 20 positive things to each other for each pesky bad one. UGH. That's what the research says. They found that if there are more bad exchanges than good, the relationship is more likely to fail. Think about this: If you talked to yourself negatively, what would happen? You would get down, get sad, depressed, maybe worse. How do we counteract that? Again, the ratio. Julia and John Gottman also talk about the "Four Horsemen," an idea based on the Four Horsemen of the Apocalypse in the Bible. The Gottmans' "horsemen" are the leading cause for breakdown and conflict in relationships. DAMN! So here they are:

1) Criticism: Blaming the other person / being judgmental. Focusing on the flaws of others.
   a. Antidote: Soft starts / warm body language – Use 'I' statements.
2) Contempt: Insults / uses put downs, mocks sarcastically, and is hostile.
   a. Antidote: Share fondness and admiration with respect and appreciation.
3) Defensiveness: Deflecting responsibility, refusing to accept feedback.
   a. Antidote: Use 'I' statements and take responsibility for your own emotions. Apologize and show remorse.
4) Stonewalling: Shutting down or going silent during important discussions.
   a. Antidote: Self-sooth! You can agree to pause the conversation while you relax and ground yourself, so you can come back and be present towards your partner.

If you practice these simple things, I swear your communication and your connection with yourself and with your relationship will be better. I recommend being curious and becoming aware of these behaviors. Maybe you do them without realizing. Play a game with each other, one where you call the other out and put a dollar in a jar, like with a swear jar, and put that money towards a trip or adventure for the two of you. This way it will lead to something positive instead of negative. Call it out by saying "HA! Horsemen!" when one is doing it. This will also bring accountability and help both of you build growth towards connection.

Or use something else that fits your relationship. That's the beauty of it; the relationship is yours, and the two of you can build it in a way that both of you can consensually agree on—because it's for you! No one else. Have fun with it! Get sexy, get proud, get into fighting fair! Say things like "I feel [about self, 'I' language here] about [current situation, no shame, blame, just state the situation naturally]" or "I need [express what you do need about it in positive way]." This can help the other understand what is happening and what your need is instead of having them try to guess. Or it can prevent finger-pointing over what isn't getting done. Author Marshall B. Rosenberg has done great work on this type of non-violent communication, or what I like to call "positive ownership."

Needless to say, with two people who have two different views, of course there is going to be some check-in chats, some noes, and some yeses. Sometimes, things might not feel completely fair in an effort to make the situation a respectful one for all parties and to create a sense of togetherness instead of individualism. We are built for connection and thrive in relationships. Basically, you won't get your way all the time. The worst is when the two of you are out of polarity, out of sync, or worse … have flat-lined. This is an indicator that you're both wanting depth and seeking it, wherever it may be. Be the one who shows up. Be the one who lights up, and be the one who owns up! However, you will make your relationship even stronger for future exploration, all while taking responsibility for yourself, which leads me to my second point: Fight fair! If you say, "I just don't want conflict or fights," get your head out of the sand and outta your ass! Things happen; out-of-your-control situations happen, which is why we learn from the crap and move forward towards a better understanding. The key to fighting fair is to hear each other, not just listen. HEAR each other. Be curious. See, really *see*, the other's point of view as well as both views. Understand fully what happened, what was going on. Do this when—you guested it—the Four Horsemen are at bay. Do not get heated and blow up! Rest, reflect, reset. The three lovely R's can help you with being logical.

Wanna deep dive more?! Read about "The Five Love Languages"** in combination with the five sex languages* to find out how you give and receive love and how you might like to give and receive pleasure!

We all know science and the brain; we've all got lots of long labels and fun words to say, but to simplify: the reasoning and logical side of the brain needs to be present in order to hear, understand, and acknowledge. This means that your emotional brain, the shit show, the hot mess that engages the Four Horsemen has to calm the eff down, wayyy down, *prior* to being able to really talk about it. Both parties need to be calm and make space for logic. Yes, it doesn't really happen 100% of the time, but think: If you start doing it, then your brain will remember ... "Oh hey, girl! Remember last time we chatted and felt heard and seen and understood during a shitty, shitty situation that happened? Want that again? Let's do that thing we did last time. It felt good!" Then BAM, that pathway is deepened. Neuropsychologist Donald Hebb says, "What fires together, wires together." He's talking about neurons developing a path after you've chosen to guide them. The more you fire that way, the more that path gets wired until it becomes the norm.

Alright, last but not least: the wonderful parties! Lots to explore, lots was done, and so much more. This came about because we had taken the time as a couple to focus on each other, and well, to be frank, we did trigger the fuck out of each other too. I came from a background of "Let's talk it out. Let's deal with it head on," and he came from a background of "Let's pretend it never happened and sweep it under the rug." As I said, we came from different backgrounds, and we worked hard and continue to work hard to unwind these beliefs and conditions that were put upon us. I had to create space, while he had to come forward. When you hear people say the biggest growth is in relationships, they are right. The reason is that nothing is hidden; your shadows, your inner being, your nooks and crannies are looked at and challenged. This doesn't just happen with intimate sexual partners. This can happen with a trustworthy friend, family member, or someone from your support network. I don't know how many times I talked it out with someone to help me calm down. Sometimes just saying something out loud and hearing it gives us the perspective we need. I came from a religious background, something that was not for me. Tristan came from a very spiritual background and broke free in his own way so he could find what called to him. Together, we have really zoned in on ourselves, and we learn from each other still.

I wanted to point out in this book moments of hardship and things that came up that aren't really talked about a lot. I wanted to point out lessons along the way and ways of exploring safely and openly. I also wanted to let readers know these aren't all the stories. We have had more-somes, twosomes, together-somes, and so on. However, the main reason for telling these stories was to show what the beginning of finding one's kink looks like, of finding one's way and navigating through it. I hope this guide helps you and helps support you in finding your inner kink!

> "To my readers,
> find your path,
> find your bounds,
> find your kink ..."
>
> – Z.

Keep exploring, keep checking in, and keep being curious with yourself and with others. Never give up on growth. Welcome your sexy inner vixen ... Let her play, grow, and shine.

Play safe, play consensually,
Zara

# Glossary

*Cock Ring*: Worn around the penis and scrotum and used for play, cock rings restrict blood flow to help a penis stay harder or fuller. This prolongs sensation, which can produce even more pleasure. However, be sure to use the correct size. If the cock ring is uncomfortable or painful, take it off immediately. P.S. There are even vibrating cock rings for ladies who want clitoral stimulation, *why hello*!

*Five Sex Languages/Erotic Blueprint*: Jaiya, a somatic sexologist, created an erotic blueprint to help others better understand themselves and each other. More details on Jaiya's erotic blueprint are available in the previous chapter or in the glossary at the back of the book under "Sensual Play."

*Fucks and Chucks*: This expression refers to fucking someone and then never speaking to them again. The experience was just to have the moment and nothing more.

*Helicopter*: When a person's penis is exposed and they swing it around to mimic helicopter blades, they are doing the "helicopter."

*Katoptronophilia*: This term is for those who experience pleasure from having sex or masturbating in front of the mirror.

*MWW:* This is the acronym for a threesome with a male, a woman, and another woman.

*Nipple Play:* This process involves playing with or licking, flicking, twisting, using clamps, straining, stroking, or teasing a person's nipples for pleasure. Yes, they are an erogenous zone, and we can have that oh-so-lovely orgasm—without even touching our genitals. There are other areas of the body that can get you off, producing that big, lovely O, besides the clitoris and vagina.

*Rim Job/Analingus:* Just as cunnilingus is to the pussy, analingus or rimming is to the asshole. This activity can be highly stimulating for some since there are lots of nerve endings there. Just make sure cleanliness is prioritized as this is most important.

*Sapiosexuality*: Finding someone attractive because of their intelligence or getting turned on by their intellect makes you a sapiosexual.

*Shakti*: In Hindu culture, the goddess counterpart of Shiva represents flow, openness, and divine changes after the raw expression of the feminine, as well as that of wisdom and creativity. The balance of Shiva and Shakti symbolizes masculine and feminine dynamics.

*Shiva*: In Hindu culture, Shiva is the god of intense, untamed passion in stillness, purpose, and masculine drive.

# EPILOGUE

To the vixens who haven't found their own way, keep on embracing your inner vixen with an open mind and an open heart. Eroticism is both internal and external.

I want to thank the ones who supported me through this, and also thank myself since, just like with this book, I pushed hard. I went through some down times and needed to take some breaks to accomplish writing it. I have a love-hate relationship with perfection because I knew the book wouldn't be perfect. It wouldn't have all the stories; the ending wouldn't be *Ahhhh* for all imaginable elements and that's ok. What I needed to do was bring it to light, to let people just read it and absorb it. Hopefully, they learn from it and learn that there is more out there than what we have all been conditioned to see. Find your own stories and embrace those boundaries as well as the gift of consent. Own your own killer worth and detach from the meaning behind things, because it may or may not be there. Embrace you!

"I'm sorry,
Please forgive me.
Thank you,
I love you,
*Ho'oponopono* (to rectify an error)."

# GLOSSARY

*ABDL*: Adult baby diaper lovers. As the name implies, ABDL involves role playing while wearing diapers, changing out of them, and so on. Fun fact—ABDL has been around a while. There is even a scholarly paper by Tuchman and Lachman, dating back to 1964. (3)

*Aftercare*: After a scene—yes, you guessed it—you care for each other (usually, the sub needs extra care). This can look like going into a separate room to check-in and cuddle, for possibly easing back into a comfy headspace to finish your scene with more even care and togetherness. Or it can mean asking for certain things or certain kinds of support. Aftercare is important because lots of chemicals release when you are highly stimulated, which in turn can cause a down/deplete later on, a.k.a. a "con drop." Things that help include rehydration/replenishment; caring for aches, pains, or marks/bruises; taking a tiny nap; check-ins/talking; and/or maybe a massage. (3, 10, 13, 18)

*Arousal Non-concordance*: Mismatched subjective (or metal) and physical arousal. Basically, your body and your mind are not on the same page sexually in that moment. (7)

*Attachment Styles:* There are four main attachment styles, which are ingrained into you basically from birth to 18 months. The first style is secure; just like it sounds, you can self-sooth, count on your caregiver to be there, and so forth. The second is an anxious attachment style, which is basically a fear of being alone. It can look like people-pleasing, low self-esteem, validation seeking, and a need to be *in the know*. The third is an avoidance or dismissive attachment style; the person is independent, distant, ambivalent, and basically uncaring if needed in a situation. This style includes a fear of intimacy, vulnerability, and commitment. The fourth is a fearful or ambivalent attachment style, which is characterized by avoidance, insecurity, poor boundaries, hot/cold personality, and—you guessed it—runs on fear. These styles were introduced by Bowlby and further developed by Ainsworth in the field of Behavioral Psychology. (11, 15)

*Ayahuasca Ceremony:* An ancient ceremony in Peru where you drink a brewed aya plant that activates DMT in your body (which is only there when you are born and dying, hence why some have a "rebirthing" experience). This should only be done by an indigenous shaman who knows the ancient ways of his culture. You will also need to pre-screen to make sure you do not do this if you have any medical conditions or are on any medication or drugs. The mother plant medicine is said to help guide you towards your growth, move you through blocks, and enlighten your understanding of the universe. It has been used to help people who have anxiety, depression, PTSD, etc. Do your research beforehand as well. (12)

*BDSM:* Bondage, discipline, dominance and submission, sadomasochism. BDSM is the term used for certain kinds of erotic play between consenting adults. Bondage is described below. Discipline is a type a punishment that is done through rule breaking or for fun. Dominance and submission are described below, as well as bottom and top. The sadomasochism* element of BDSM represents the act of deriving pleasure by giving or receiving pain, torture, or humiliation. (3, 4, 10, 18)

*Bi-curious:* A heterosexual person who is interested in sexual experiences with a person of the same sex. This could be in a fantasy context, play context, or another context. (14)

*Bi-situational:* A heterosexual person who is interested in sexual experiences with another person of the same gender, depending on the circumstances and situation, a.k.a. "mostly straight." (14)

*Bisexual:* Those who identify as bisexual feel a sexual and/or romantic attraction to people of a different gender or of the same gender. This term gets tossed around a lot, even for those who are only bi-curious. A.K.A. "Bi." (14)

*Body-Positivity:* An attitude or approach in which people are free to express themselves in how they dress; free to be any shape, size, gender, orientation; free from judgment and discrimination; essentially, your body, your choice; absolutely no shaming. (11)

*Bondage:* In BDSM subculture, bondage is the practice of tying, binding, or restraining someone consensually. (3)

*Bottom:* This term is used to refer to a certain sexual or psychological preference for the role of the submissive or passive. This does not necessarily mean the person is sexually on the bottom. (3)

*Boundaries:* Where you end and the other begins; what you're ok and not ok with. (3,4,7,9,10,11,13,14,15,16,17,18)

*Brat:* In the lifestyle/kink community, "brat" is a term used when someone wants to be put in their place by a master, Dom, or tamer.

Brats act out almost like teenagers and receive "punishments" in return. Most importantly, this is all consensual. (10)

*Breath Play*: This type of play seeks to restrict someone's breathing for the purpose of pleasure. (17)

*Chlamydia:* A sexually transmitted disease that is more common than some would think. There may be no symptoms, or there may be discharge and/or a burning sensation while peeing and/or swelling. Best to ask your doctor and get checked. And use protection! (15)

*Cock Ring*: Worn around the penis and scrotum and used for play, cock rings restrict blood flow to help a penis stay harder or fuller. This prolongs sensation, which can produce even more pleasure. However, be sure to use the correct size. If the cock ring is uncomfortable or painful, take it off immediately. P.S. There are even vibrating cock rings for ladies who want clitoral stimulation, why hello! (18)

*Compersion*: This quality is well known in the lifestyle or BDSM/kink community. The opposite of jealousy, compersion allows you to experience pleasure from seeing your partner get pleasure. (17)

*The Corkscrew*: Use your hand up the shaft, going to the top, then gripping at the bottom again and twist—with lube—gently, with slight pressure up, and repeat. For more on blowjobs, a good book is *Heads Up: Increase your sexual confidence, expand your sexual repertoire, and get the real lowdown on oral sex* by Dr. Teesha Morgan and Constance Lynn Hummel. (13)

*Cuckolding*: With this kink, your partner loves watching you have sex with another person. Seeing you get pleasure, knowing they're going to get it as well, turns them on. Cuckolding is done of course with the consent of all parties involved. And it is not as uncommon as you would think. (17)

*DDLG or Daddy Dom/Little Girl Play*: This kind of play involves consenting adults who may or may not dress up. They satisfy each other's needs by giving/getting the care and attention they need/crave. Dom daddies exert positive masculinity (and mommies exert a nurturing femininity). A "little" acts as if they are a child. (3)

*Dom*: Persons who take a "dominant" role are Doms (male) or Dommes (female). (3, 6, 9)

*Dominatrix*: A woman who takes the "dominant" role in BDSM activities. One who takes the lead. (6, 18)

*DP (Double Penetration)*: Usually, this involves one woman consenting to penetration from one guy from the front (vagina) and one penetrating her from the back (butt), a.k.a. "One in the pink and one in the stink," but—that expression sucks, so please don't use it. (10)

*Dungeon Master a.k.a. Dungeon Monitor*: a person who monitors the play space. To make sure consent is followed, there are safe sex practices, as well as a designated person to come to if there is an issue. Dungeon masters (or monitors) are clearly indicated, usually by tag, introduction, or uniform. (4, 9)

*DV (Double Vagina)*: DV happens when a woman takes two cocks in the pussy at the same time. DP is sometimes used in lieu of DV. (10)

*Edgeplay or Edging*: In BDSM, edgeplay or edging means riding the edge. However, edgeplay focuses on the psychological mindfuck and on expanding what you think you can handle, while edging focuses on riding the edge of an orgasm. You can do this with breathing, being present, slowing down, or taking breaks. Edging can prolong your orgasm, produce a more powerful orgasm, or help you enjoy the journey and sensation of being in the moment. (3, 18)

*Eiffel Tower / Going to Paris*: In this instance, we did MMF (two males and one female). The woman is on all fours and in between the two guys. She sucks one of the guys off while the other one pounds her from behind, then the two guys high-five. Without the high-fives, apparently, this position is called a split roast, which isn't a very sexy name, but comes from the view of the person in the middle being "skewered." Needless to say, thank God for high-fives! (17)

*Electrical Play*: This type of play usually involves a wand**, with attachments that can be adjusted according to your desired strength. The wand is a medical device from the Victorian era that is now used as a sex toy and/or for edgeplay** or edging and stimulation. (3)

*Exhibitionist*: An exhibitionist likes putting on a show for others, and they get aroused by doing so. Usually, exhibitionism is consensual, and it is often associated with voyeurism, which occurs when someone becomes aroused by watching others put on a show. Voyeurism is also usually consensual. (4, 8, 17)

*Femmey/ Femme*: In this context, the male bringing out his feminine role, with more feminine aspects. Such as wearing female lingerie, wigs, being more submissive, etc. Embodies and embraces the feminine through sexy empowerment.

*Fantasize*: We often dream or daydream about things we might be longing to try. The key here is that fantasizing doesn't mean you actually want the fantasy to happen; fantasizing is your mind wandering all over the place and going over taboo possibilities it wants to play out! Yes, I'm talking about sexual fantasies here. Consent is necessary when you actually do want to see a fantasy through, as well as having that good ol' boundary chat and establishing a safe word. For example, you might want to explore a sexual rape fantasy where saying no is part of the fantasy, but you will need a certain word, agreed upon ahead of time, to use if you need to call a complete stop to the situation. When does fantasy become a tad unhealthy? When it affects your daily life and you are constantly longing for what you're fantasizing about. Most fantasies are just that—fantasies. (5)

*Fetish*: To have a fetish is to enjoy a nonsexual object or body part sexually. Common fetishes include feet and shoes, leather, or rubber. (3, 11, 14, 16, 18,)

*Fight, Flight, or Freeze Response*: When your lovely body activates its fight, flight, or freeze response, it is attempting to protect you from danger. This survival mechanism prompts you to either escape, fight for your life, or freeze so as to be ignored or not "seen." In BDSM play, this response can either help you or hold you back. There is another option referred to as "fawn," in which a sub basically agrees to whatever the Dom decrees in order to save themselves. (4)

*Fire Play*: Here, alcohol was set on fire on the skin. This BDSM practice is exactly what the name implies—playing with fire in a safe manner. Every time I have had friends do fire play, safety measures, such as a fire extinguisher—were always present. (3)

*Flogger*: A flogger is a BDSM/kink toy that is used to "flog" someone. Flogging is a type of impact play** that involves technique, and the range of sensation can go from light and sensual to thudding or stinging, depending on what the players desire and discuss beforehand. In a non-BDSM context, you can also see floggers used for horses. They are made out of leather with a handle at one end. (3, 16, 18)

*Fucks and Chucks*: This expression refers to fucking someone and then never speaking to them again. The experience was just to have the moment and nothing more. (18)

*Furry Fetish:* Getting turned on by dressing up in an animal costume, still with human capabilities. (14)

*G-spot*: This area is located two to three inches inside a woman's vagina, usually up the front of the vaginal wall, between the vaginal opening and the urethra. You know you have hit the "spot" when you feel a soft, squishy, almost sponge-like texture. This well-known spot got its "G" from a German gynecologist named Ernest Gräfenberg in 1981. (17, 18)

*Helicopter*: When a person's penis is exposed and they swing it around to mimic helicopter blades, they are doing the "helicopter." (18)

*Impact Play*: This is a type of play that involves using toys or instruments for pain that is pleasurable. It can be a huge turn-on, and consent, of course, is a must. (17)

*Intersex*: A person born with both reproductive or sexual parts, an intersex person doesn't classify themselves as "male" or "female." (10)

*Katoptronophilia*: This term is for those who experience pleasure from having sex or masturbating in front of the mirror. (18)

*Kava Ceremony:* An ancient ceremony where you sit in a circle in front of the leader or group facilitator, and you communicate your intentions and gratitude and all drink at once (this is how we did it). Kava root is known for its power to connect to the soul and for promoting relaxation naturally. It can make your tongue tingle a bit. (14)

*Kegels*: This exercise helps women strengthen their pelvic floor muscles. Kegels can also improve sexual function and treat incontinence. The exercise involves repeatedly contracting and relaxing your pelvic floor muscles; some people use a jade egg (sometimes referred to as a yoni egg) or other device to help with this. (16)

*Kink*: Something that brings you pleasure/turns you on but also bends away from the "straight and narrow." You could have a kink for bondage, whips, chains, dress up, role play, or something more subtle. Kinks are usually considered non-conventional sexual practices. (1, 3, 8, 9, 11, 13, 14, 17, 18)

*Kinksters*: People who enjoy kinky things or kinks. (3)

*London Bridge*: This position is a combination of the superhero, the asteroid, and the bridge. The woman is on her back, her legs pointing towards the ceiling, and a guy pounds her between the legs, while another holds her legs (could be one or two people). The woman or the guy or guys holding her legs is/are free to fondle any of the others, whatever everyone is up for. (17)

*Love Languages*: In "The Five Love Languages," a book by Gary Chapman, the "love languages" include words of affirmation, quality time, physical touch, acts of service, and receiving gifts. You can take a test online that will tell you which of the love languages you "speak" the best (ranked by percentage), and this information can be used to improve your relationship. For example, if I like physical touch, but my partner like words of affirmation, then their love language may mean telling me how beautiful and sexy I am, and mine means I prefer giving my partner a back massage. When the other person knows where you stand, you can both understand each other's own way of expressing love. (10, 17, 18)

*Low Tails*: This accessory usually indicates that a person is wearing a butt plug with a tail attached. (11)

*Masochism*: The practice of deriving sexual pleasure from pain; a masochist is one who gets turned on by being hurt. (8)

*Master*: A master is the one who calls the shots, with the consent of the submissive person who calls them such. Masters are often dominant and stern. (9, 10, 11, 18)

*MWW:* This is the acronym for a threesome with a male, a woman, and another woman.

*Monogamish:* This is a great term for people who aren't quite monogamous or non-monogamous. These couples kind of dabble on the edge and play within or dip their toe in some light, non-monogamous flirtatious play and toy with the idea with their partner. This idea comes around when going to certain events or maybe putting on a show or telling their partner certain wild things they would like to do with others, etc. but not actually doing it. However, there are different definitions of this, and I believe in creating a relationship based on what relationship you want to create together and not defining it based on a label. (5)

*Munches:* These are social gatherings for BDSM, kink, or lifestyle people to gather under relaxed settings. They usually happen at a restaurant, bar, lunch spot, or over coffee. The goal is to find like-minded people and connect to the community. (3)

*Nipple Play:* This process involves playing with or licking, flicking, twisting, using clamps, straining, stroking, or teasing a person's nipples for pleasure. Yes, they are an erogenous zone, and we can have that oh-so-lovely orgasm—without even touching our genitals. There are other areas of the body that can get you off, producing that big, lovely O, besides the clitoris and vagina.

*OM:* Orgasmic meditation is a practice of nest building, one-way touch or fully receiving every sensation. The touch is a mindful pleasure in which the giver uses a certain technique with the receiver, like playing a violin. OM usually lasts around 15 minutes, and it involves slow, consistent, but small—barely touching! —strokes of the clitoris. I bet you haven't heard about that one! And yes, it can he healing and a full-blown release! (14)

*Orgasmic Control*: This practice involves controlling yourself from orgasming by stopping or slowing down, usually with breathing, and then bringing yourself back to the peak. (17)

*Pegging*: A sexual practice in which a woman performs anal sex on a man by penetrating his anus with a strap-on dildo. (6)

*Play:* A term I use that includes everything up to oral, but not penis-in-vagina. "Play" could mean different things for different people, so ask! (1, 3, 6, 7, 8, 9, 10, 11, 12, 13, 14, 15, 16, 17, 18)

*Play Partner*: A play partner is someone who may or may not be a person's primary partner. A play partner is someone you scene or play out a fetish with. The scene does not usually include penetration but can if discussed beforehand and consent is given. (3)

*Polyamorous*: a.k.a. "poly" or "polyam" is a type of non-monogamous relationship dynamic. One or both partners may desire to be intimate with more than one person, while still maintaining the primary relationship, with their partner's informed consent. More people are leaning towards ethical non-monogamy (ENM) since it's becoming less taboo and more mainstream. There is discussion about replacing the term "poly" with "polyam," since "poly" can sometimes be used to refer to Polynesian people. (10)

*Puppy Play or Pup Play*: This term is for a situation in which one person takes the role of a pup, while the other one takes the on role of a handler, consensually of course. (1)

*Rigger*: A riggers ties (a) person(s) up in a sexual kink/BDSM context. The rigging can vary from ceiling hooks to crosses. This player is very aware and focused on the play partner that they are tying. They are also very skilled and will have discussed safety, safe words, and the play partner's needs with the play partner. This knowledge will allow them to focus on the tension of the whole experience as well as on expressing their mastery and on recognizing if something isn't working. (3)

*Rim Job/Analingus*: Just as cunnilingus is to the pussy, analingus or rimming is to the asshole. This activity can be highly stimulating for some since there are lots of nerve endings there. Just make sure cleanliness is prioritized as this is most important. (18)

*Safe Word*: A word, usually other than "no," that indicates a stop to everything and/or that a check-in is needed. This can also be a gesture or something you do, such as dropping something in order to signal to a play partner that they need to stop. Sometimes, words won't compute or are limited by a gag or some other element in a scene. (1, 3, 11)

*Sapiosexuality*: Finding someone attractive because of their intelligence or getting turned on by their intellect makes you a sapiosexual.

*Sassafras:* A pure form of drug extracted from a rare plant. The sensation resembles that of being on molly. Molly is MDMA, which is a chemical of sensory input that dumps feel-good receptors—serotonin, dopamine, and norepinephrine. (15)

*Scene*: A time when a BDSM/kink/lifestyle activity occurs; includes different types of play that are discussed beforehand. (3, 4, 7, 10, 11, 18)

*Scene Blues*: Low moments that might feel like regret or an energy dip after a scene happens. (7)

*Sensual Play*: This form of erotic pleasure makes you horny with light touch/massaging. "Sensual" is one of five erotic blueprints founded by somatic sexologist Jaiya. The other erotic blueprints are energetic, sexual, kinky, and shapeshifter. This idea is similar to that of the five love languages**, but for intimacy and pleasure. Jaiya created the five blueprints to help others better understand themselves and each other. (17, 18)

*Sex-Positive*: Normalizing sexuality for pleasure as a consent culture. (4, 8, 11, 18)

*Sexual/Erotic Asphyxiation*: This sexual practice is a kind of breath play** in which one intentionally restricts their or their partner's oxygen by chocking, hanging, or other means. Erotic asphyxiation is a BDSM term under the umbrella term of "breath play." This kind of play can be dangerous so be mindful; there have been deaths related to erotic asphyxiation. (17)

*Sexual Compliance*: There might be times when you say yes to a sexual partner even if you don't particularly feel like having sex. The reason you might comply sexually when you don't necessarily want to are complex and varied. (7)

*Sexual Massage:* Involves one-way touch as the masseuse only touches you. This touch is whole-body and does not exclude any part of the body unless discussed ahead of time. Sexual massage is used to help overcome sexual trauma through safe, consensual touch. It is slow, soft, and sensual but includes some pressure. A full-body orgasm or just an orgasm can happen. Sounds are encouraged to express pleasure. (14)

*Sexual Polarity*: Occurs when masculine and feminine dynamics are in sync with each other in perfect harmony or pleasure. Energy entwines the two as if nothing else matters—no thoughts, only the senses, pleasure, and oneness. David Deida says in his book *Intimate Communion*, "Sexual polarity—the magnetic pull or repulsion between the Masculine and Feminine—affects all our lives." (12, 13, 15, 16, 18)

*Shakti*: In Hindu culture, the goddess counterpart of Shiva represents flow, openness, and divine changes after the raw expression of the feminine, as well as that of wisdom and creativity. The balance of Shiva and Shakti symbolizes masculine and feminine dynamics. (18)

*Shibari*: Ancient Japanese rope play, bondage. (3)

*Shiva*: In Hindu culture, Shiva is the god of intense, untamed passion in stillness, purpose, and masculine drive. (18)

*Sir*: "Sir" is a BDSM term that two parties can choose to use in their relationship (either while playing in a scene or all the time, depending on the relationship). "Sir" is most often used in reference to or when addressing the dominant partner; however, sirs are typically gentler than a master. Other common terms for the dominant include: Master/Mistress, Dom/Domme, or Top. (10, 18)

*SOP*: Sex on the premises. (4, 11)

*Squirting*: During orgasm/ejaculation, a woman can expel fluid. Some say it is a deep release, almost as if they've peed; some report it as an overflow of fluid; and some don't even know what happened until it did. Don't be discouraged; not everyone can squirt, and that's ok. Also, squirting can be messy so better have lots of towels on board. (17, 18)

*St. Andrew's Cross*: This type of cross is shaped like an "X." These types of crosses allow for tying, flogging, playing, blindfolding, or whatever the sub/Dom wants to play around with. A St. Andrew's cross is usually leather bound with tie-down rings on four or more points. Its name refers to a story in which Saint Andrew was said to have been martyred by crucifixion. (3, 7, 12, 18)

*Starfish*: A sexual position where one essentially lies like a starfish, wide open in the missionary position as a bottom, hands and legs spread so the other person has to do all the work. (8)

*STIs*: Sexually transmitted diseases, yay! Not really. They are caused by one person passing on a bacteria, virus, or parasite to another, either during sex or intimate contact. It is best to use protection like condoms when engaging in sexual activities. Some of the most common STIs are: Chlamydia, Gonorrhea, Hepatitis B (HBV), Herpes (HSV-1, HSV-2), Genital warts/Human Papillomavirus (HPV) infection, and Syphilis. For more information, you can always do a good ol' Google search on a reputable site, such as the Mayo Clinic or the Center for Disease Control in your area. (2)

*Sub*: Persons who take the subordinate position are called "submissive" or "subs" (male or female). (3, 6, 9, 10)

*Suspension*: Suspension occurs when you're tied up and off the ground, suspended in air with rope. (3)

*Swingers*: Couples who have consensual sexual relations with other couples. (9, 13)

*Switch*: A switch goes back and forth between two preferences, usually bottom and top and depending on the scene. (3, 18)

*Sybian machine:* A device you ride on that has different attachments with different speeds. Usually used for female masturbation, it can be for oral play and a fun way for couples to experiment with the speed dial. (9, 18)

*The Sex Show*: This "upscale" adult playground is dedicated to enhancing the lifestyle, encouraging romance, personal betterment, and all things taboo. This is usually accomplished through demonstrations, intimacy trinkets, promoting sex workers, pole dancing, kink, introductions to BDSM, prizes, and art. (17)

*Tantra:* In Sanskrit, the word "tantra" means "woven together," and the aim is to achieve mindfulness and deep connection for its participants through breathwork, extended eye contact, embraces, massages, and slow, present intercourse. Tantra can occur with or without sex. Involves energy work. (14)

*Top*: This term is used to refer to a certain sexual or psychological preference for the role of the dominant or active partner when playing. This does not necessarily mean the person is sexually on top. NOTE: This definition is different for gay men. Please be mindful. Different definitions can mean different things for different people, so it's best to ask what their version is. (3)

*Vanilla*: This term refers to people who are monogamous, or those who aren't familiar with kink, fetish, or lifestyle worlds. "Vanilla" could also be used for people who are new to the scene. (11)

*Wand a.k.a. the violet wand*: This device uses an Oudin coil to apply low-current, high-voltage electricity to the body. The wand has medical benefits and is also used in sadomasochistic** sex play. (3)

# BOOKS

Kink/Sex/Lifestyle:

1. *Leading and Supportive Love: The Truth About Dominant and Submissive Relationships* by Chris M. Lyon
2. *Playing Well with Others: Your Field Guide to Discovering, Exploring and Navigating the Kink, Leather and BDSM Communities* by Lee Harrington and Mollena Williams
3. *Polysecure: Attachment, Trauma and Consensual Nonmonogamy* by Jessica Fern
4. *The Ethical Slut: A Practical Guide to Polyamory, Open Relationships & Other Adventures* by Janet W. Hardy and Dossie Easton (older now)
5. *She Comes First: The Thinking Man's Guide to Pleasuring a Woman* by Ian Kerner
6. *Heads Up: Increase your sexual confidence, expand your sexual repertoire, and get the real lowdown on oral sex* by Dr. Teesha Morgan and Constance Lynn Hummel
7. *Come As You Are: The Surprising New Science that Will Transform Your Sex Life* by Emily Nagoski
8. *Desire: The Tantric Path to Awakening* by Daniel Odier
9. *Sex at Dawn: The Prehistoric Origins of Modern Sexuality* by Christopher Ryan

10. *Women's Anatomy of Arousal: Secret Maps to Buried Pleasure* by Sheri Winston
11. *The Erotic Mind: Unlocking the Inner Sources of Passion* by Jack Morin
12. *Pussy: A Reclamation* by Regena Thomashauer
13. *Topping* By Dossie Easton and Janet Hardy,
14. *Bottoming* By Janet W. Hardy and Dossie Easton,
15. *Ultimate Guide to Kink: BDSM, Role Play and The Erotic Edge* by Tristan Taormino

Spiritual/Relationship:

1. *The Way of the Superior Man: A Spiritual Guide to Mastering the Challenges of Women, Work, and Sexual Desire* by David Deida
2. *Intimate Communion: Awakening Your Sexual Essence* by David Deida
3. *The Mindful Couple: How Acceptance and Mindfulness Can Lead You to the Love You Want* by Robyn D. Walser and Darrah Westrup
4. *Eight Dates: Essential Conversations for a Lifetime of Love* by John Gottman and Julie Schwartz Gottman
5. *Keys to the Kingdom* by Alison A. Armstrong
6. *The 5 Love Languages* by Gary Chapman
7. *Attached: Are you Anxious, Avoidant or Secure? How the science of adult attachment can help you find – and keep – love* by Amir Levine and Rachel Heller
8. *In Sync with the Opposite Sex* by Alison A. Armstrong
9. *The New Codependency: Help and Guidance for Today's Generation* by Melody Beattie and Lorna Raver
10. *Mating in Captivity: Unlocking Erotic Intelligence* by Esther Perel

11. *The Jewel in the Lotus/The Tantric Path to Higher Consciousness* by Bodhi Avinasha
12. *The Seven Spiritual Laws of Success* by Deepak Chopra

Self-Exploration:

1. *Daring Greatly: How the Courage to Be Vulnerable Transforms the Way We Live, Love, Parent, and Lead* by Brené Brown
2. *The Four Agreements: A Practical Guide to Personal Freedom* by Don Miguel Ruiz
3. *The Subtle Art of Not Giving a Fuck* by Mark Manson
4. *The Six Pillars of Self-Esteem* by Nathaniel Branden
5. *Beyond Mars and Venus: Relationship Skills for Today's Complex World* by John Gray
6. *The Language of Letting Go: Daily Meditations for Codependents* by Melody Beattie
7. *You Are a Badass: How to Stop Doubting Your Greatness and Start Living an Awesome Life* by Jen Sincero
8. *Dare to Lead* by Brené Brown
9. *Nonviolent Communication: A Language of Life* by Marshall B. Rosenberg
10. *The Anxiety Toolkit: Strategies for Fine-Tuning Your Mind and Moving Past Your Stuck Points* by Alice Boyes
11. *Transcendent CEO* by Satyen Raja
12. *Molecules of Emotion: The Science Behind Mind-Body Medicine* by Candace B. Pert

Trauma:

1. *The Complex PTSD Workbook: A Mind-Body Approach to Regaining Emotional Control and Becoming Whole* by Arielle Schwartz

2. *In the Realm of Hungry Ghosts: Close Encounters with Addiction* by Gabor Maté
3. *How to Do the Work: Recognize Your Patterns, Heal from Your Past, and Create Your Self* by Nicole LePera
4. *The Body Keeps the Score: Brain, Mind, and Body in the Healing of Trauma* by Bessel van der Kolk
5. *No Bad Parts: Healing Trauma and Restoring Wholeness with the Internal Family Systems Model* by Richard Schwartz

# ABOUT THE AUTHOR

Well known in the lifestyle community, Zara Fox is constantly exploring lifestyle destinations and events internationally. She wanted to write this book on how to overcome the challenges that may arise and also share her experiences to hopefully help others navigate through tough situations.

Now that Tristan and Zara have fully embraced their relationship, don't miss them embracing it beyond—with *Destinations* ...

CPSIA information can be obtained
at www.ICGtesting.com
Printed in the USA
BVHW080458011222
653162BV00016B/273